MAJOR PROBLEMS IN INTERNAL MEDICINE

In Preparation

DAVID G. COGAN, M.D.

Henry Willard Williams Professor of Ophthalmology, Emeritus
Director of the Howe Laboratory of Ophthalmology
Harvard Medical School
Medical Officer, United States Public Health Service

OPHTHALMIC MANIFESTATIONS OF SYSTEMIC VASCULAR DISEASE

VOLUME

III

IN THE SERIES
MAJOR PROBLEMS IN INTERNAL MEDICINE

Lloyd H. Smith, Jr., M. D., *Editor*

W. B. SAUNDERS COMPANY • PHILADELPHIA • LONDON • TORONTO • 1974

W. B. Saunders Company: West Washington Square
                           Philadelphia, Pa. 19105

                           12 Dyott Street
                           London, WC1A   1DB

                           W. B. Saunders Company Canada Ltd.
                           833 Oxford Street
                           Toronto, Ontario M8Z 5T9, Canada

Cogan, David Glendenning, 1908–

Ophthalmic manifestations of systemic vascular disease.

(Major problems in internal medicine, v. 3)

Includes bibliographical references.

1. Ocular manifestations of general diseases.

2. Blood-vessels — Diseases.   I. Title. [DNLM: 1. Eye
   manifestations.   2. Vascular diseases — Diagnosis.
   WI MA492T v.3 / WG500 C675o]

RE65.C63   616.1′3′072   74–4556

ISBN 0–7216–2648–3

Ophthalmic Manifestations of Systemic Vascular Disease   ISBN 0-7216-2648-3

Last digit is the print number: 9   8   7   6   5   4   3   2   1

FOREWORD

There are two organ systems which are readily examined by direct visualization, the skin and the eye. The skin is uniquely available for gross examination. It can be more readily biopsied for microscopic study than can any other tissue except for the blood. Cell lines of skin fibroblasts can be established in tissue culture for sophisticated studies of metabolic disorders in vitro. Because of these attributes, the skin readily serves as a mirror for a large variety of systemic illnesses. There are limitations, however, in using the skin as an index tissue for direct examination. In order to be protective, it must be tough, relatively thick, and opaque. Most of its structures cannot, therefore, be readily examined in life.

The eye, on the other hand, is admirably adapted to direct examination. The structures which admit light to stimulate the retina, an exteriorized portion of the central nervous system, can equally transmit light back to the eye of the observer. In a sense, vision allows visualization. Nowhere else can the structures of an organ be so readily examined during life. This holds particularly true for the vascular system. The whole arborization of arteries, capillaries, and veins can be examined in the retina and in the scleral conjunctiva. In this monograph, Dr. David G. Cogan has summarized current knowledge concerning normal and abnormal vasculature so revealed in examination of the eye. In this treatment of a complex subject, he has furnished a rational approach to the evaluation of abnormal states and has illustrated these states with informative examples in more than 100 photographs. As Professor of Ophthalmology at Harvard Medical School and Director of the Howe Laboratory of Ophthalmology, Dr. Cogan has worked closely with all of the clinical departments at the Massachusetts General Hospital for many years in pursuing his special interest in ophthalmology as a branch of general medicine. This book reflects that breadth of interest and experience. It is most appropriate that it be published in a series entitled "Major Problems in Internal Medicine." The information presented here so lucidly and succinctly is directly pertinent to the practice of internal medicine.

LLOYD H. SMITH, JR., M.D.

PREFACE

The aim of this brief text is to provide an introduction to the always fascinating but sometimes complex relationship of the eye to vascular disease. The eye's transparent media offer a unique opportunity for direct visualization of the vessels, and ophthalmology's instrumentation enables precise means for their examination.

Blood vessels in the conjunctiva are typical of those in connective tissue elsewhere but have the great advantage of availability for examination during life, and this with microscopic magnification. Blood vessels of the retina are, on the other hand, typical of those seen in the brain but are also accessible for examination during life, although with usually less than microscopic magnification. The information that can be gleaned from these examinations, and from neuro-ophthalmic examination, has immense practical importance. Yet the observations are still largely in the descriptive stage. This text testifies, therefore, as much to ignorance as to knowledge.

The practical aspects of the eye's morbid vascular system are the dominant theme in the present composition. Only such morphology and physiology are presented as would enhance the understanding of disease. Some chapters stress signs and symptoms while other chapters stress disease entities. In this way it is hoped to serve the interest of physicians who may wish to refer either to the manifestations of disease or to the diseases themselves.

The amount of literature relevant to vascular disease and the eye is overwhelming and my citations can serve only as an introduction to source material. I have tried to credit original observations and to note authorities for controversial opinions, with, admittedly, a personal bias.

Some of the illustrations have been previously published in the following journals or systems: American Journal of Ophthalmology, Archives of Ophthalmology, British Journal of Ophthalmology, and Medcom, Inc. This latter contains some of the fundus pictures in the form of kodachrome slides.

For the preparation of this text I have had the assistance of many persons whom it is a pleasure to acknowledge: Dr. David D. Donaldson, who took most of the fundus photographs; Dr. Toichiro Kuwabara, who prepared and photographed many of the microscopic sections; Miss Marsha Jessup, who did the art work; Mrs. Maria Churchwell, who assisted in the reference search; and especially my assistants, Ms. Marjorie Saunders, Carole Hardy, and May Vuilleumier, who organized and typed several versions of the manuscript, hunted references, and relieved me of the many chores which plague a book-writer. To them and to my wife, who allowed my work top priority, I am deeply grateful.

DAVID G. COGAN

CONTENTS

Chapter 3

SIGNIFICANCE OF FUNDUS SIGNS

Chapter 4

SUBJECTIVE SYMPTOMS AND VISUAL FIELD ABNORMALITIES

Chapter 5

FUNDUS SIGNS OF SYSTEMIC VASCULAR DISEASE

Chapter 9

NEURO-OPHTHALMIC COMPLICATIONS OF INTRACRANIAL
VASCULAR DISEASE

CHAPTER 1

EXTERNAL OCULAR SIGNS

METHODS OF EXAMINATION

Gross inspection of the eye can give some indication of vascular disease or of disease mediated through the vascular system. Thus, the yellow color of the sclera may be the first indication of jaundice, and a porcelain appearance suggests anemia. Conjunctival petechiae indicate a hemorrhagic diathesis or circulatory stasis at the capillary or paracapillary level.[533] Blood-borne chemicals may produce such characteristic discoloration as the grayness of argyrosis after prolonged ingestion of silver salts or the duskiness of chrysiasis after continued administration of gold medication. Pigment deposits in the conjunctiva are characteristic of alkaptonuria. Lipemia induces a lactescence in the vessels,[186] and circulatory failure manifests a detectable cyanosis. These are a few examples of what a superficial examination of the eye may suggest.

The slit-lamp biomicroscope is most useful in studying patients with hyperviscosity syndromes or patients with morphologic changes in their small blood vessels. The biomicroscope is a low-power (5 to 20 ×) binocular microscope racked horizontally and fitted with a slit illuminating light; hence the common designation, slit-lamp microscope. It provides sufficient magnification for visualization of the conjunctival circulation in vivo. The arterial flow is usually too rapid to be seen but the capillary flow is easily perceived as clumps of red blood cells moving in a continuous or intermittent stream. The continuity and speed of this flow will vary with the heat of the examining light and the manipulation of the lids as well as with hemodynamic factors. The circulation is characteristically slow and intermittent ("sludged")[390, 391, 526] in such hyperviscosity syndromes as polycythemia and dysglobulinemia and in stenosis of the afferent vessels.

1

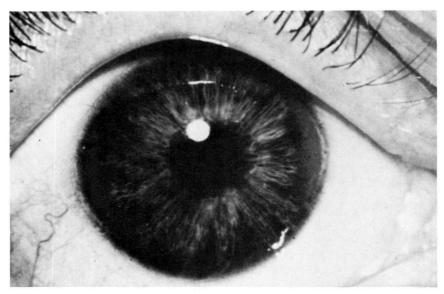

Figure 1 Band keratopathy with hypercalcemia. Significant is the grayish opacity forming an arc within the palpebral fissure at the left side of the cornea. It is not to be confused with the white (nonspecific) line peripheral to it and separating it from the limbus.

The patient was a middle-aged woman whose hypercalcemia resulted from excessive vitamin D intake.

The biomicroscope has been extensively used in attempts to correlate morphologic changes in the conjunctival blood vessels with those of arteriosclerosis,[132, 480] hypertension, Raynaud's disease,[466] and diabetes[152, 154, 232, 459] but the normal variation is so great as to limit the clinical usefulness of most of these observations (see p. 12).[213] The biomicroscope is indispensable, however, for detection in the conjunctiva and cornea of such crystalline deposits as occur with cystinosis,[75, 113, 234] dysproteinemia,[17, 526] and chlorpromazine medication.[143] The slit lamp is also useful in detecting the early deposits of calcium in the cornea[104, 108] and conjunctiva[405, 667, 698] with hypercalcemia. The corneal deposit occurs in the paralimbal region of the palpebral fissure (Fig. 1) and thereby constitutes one form of band keratopathy, but it requires a sophisticated observer to differentiate minor changes from the nonspecific calcification which also occurs in the paralimbal region.

The band keratopathy of hypercalcemia differs from that which occurs in degenerating eyes, rheumatoid arthritis, uveitis, and without apparent cause in that the calcium is deposited preferentially in the axial region with these conditions rather than in the periphery. Moreover, it differs from the common limbal calcification of age (the "limbal girdle") in being a gray deposit with small lacunae where minute plaques have sloughed off rather than the jagged white lines beneath the limbal epithelium.

Band keratopathy with calcific deposits in the cornea and conjunctiva may also occur in uremia accompanied by a low or normal serum calcium but with elevated serum phosphorous. In such cases the Ca × P quotient exceeds 70.[53, 290]

The primary use of the slit-lamp biomicroscope by ophthalmologists is for studying the following: the anterior segment of eye, the regularity of the corneal surfaces, infiltration of the corneal stroma, inflammatory cells in the anterior chambers, abnormalities of the iris, and opacities of the lens. It may also be used by experienced observers (with the auxiliary use of a contact glass) for viewing the fundus.

CONGESTION AND THE RED EYE

The red eye syndrome incorporates several entities which, although having in common dilatation of vessels, are usually distinguishable by their gross appearances. All are important in considering the etiologic interpretation of congestive phenomena.

Inflammation

Inflammatory conditions are usually characterized by a dilatation of all the vessels but predominantly of the fine vessels. With conjunctivitis this varies, according to its severity, from mild dilatation of the vessels arising in the periphery to a fiery red suffusion of the entire conjunctiva. With keratitis and iridocyclitis, on the other hand, the perilimbal and deeper vessels are preferentially involved, with consequent bluish red discoloration about the cornea. (A further point of differentiation is, of course, the purulent discharge with the former and the watery discharge with the latter.)

Passive Congestion

Passive congestion, in contrast to inflammatory congestion, causes dilatation of a few large vessels that overlie the sclera. These are veins, some coming from the periphery but some emerging abruptly through scleral channels from the interior of the eye (Fig. 2).

Passive congestion may occur nonspecifically with orbital masses, especially those involving the extraocular muscles, and is especially frequent with congestive dysthyroid exophthalmos. Passive congestion also occurs, sometimes prominently, with the various hyperviscosity syndromes, including macroglobulinemia, multiple myeloma,

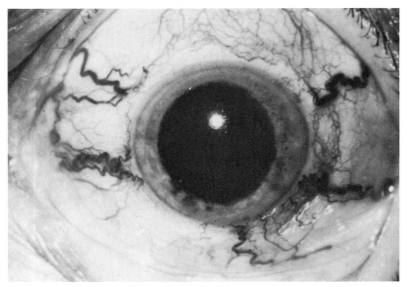

Figure 2   Passive congestion of conjunctival and episcleral vessels. Characteristic of congestion is the predominant engorgement of a few large vessels emerging abruptly in the perilimbal region and coursing sinuously to the periphery of the conjunctiva.

The patient was a 70 year old woman with bilateral exophthalmus presumed to be due to dysthyroidism.

leukemia, and polycythemia. The redness is sometimes mistaken for conjunctivitis.[19]

Active Congestion

Active congestion is a term that may be applied to those conditions in which the artery contributes primarily to the congestion. It includes especially the congestion accompanying cavernous sinus fistulas and that with selective stenosis of the internal carotid artery.

The cavernous sinus fistulas result from either rupture of a carotid artery aneurysm into the cavernous sinus (Fig. 3) or from the formation of a shunt between one of the dural vessels and the cavernous sinus (Fig. 4; also see p. 145). In either case the venous lake becomes subjected to arterial pressure and causes back-up in the orbit (pulsating exophthalmos) and congestion of the conjunctival and episcleral vessels.

The ocular congestion which occurs with stenosis of an internal carotid artery is due to the development of a bypass by way of the external carotid artery.[214] Unable to reach the brain by way of the internal carotid, blood from the common carotid passes up to the orbit through the external carotid and enters the cranium by reverse flow in the ophthalmic artery (see p. 110). In the process the conjunctival ves-

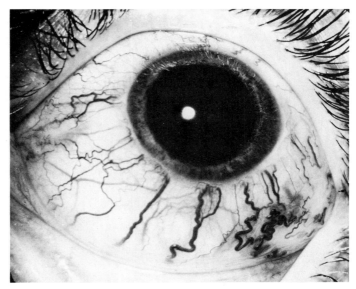

Figure 3   Active congestion resulting from a carotid-cavernous sinus fistula.

The patient was a 22 year old man whose fistula resulted from a skull fracture consequent to an automobile accident.

sels which are normally supplied by the external carotid become dilated (Fig. 5), and the lid may show a pseudoptosis from vascular stasis.

This obstruction of the internal carotid artery contrasts with obstruction of the common carotid artery in which there may be a *decreased* flow in the conjunctival vessels and a paucity of minute vessels.[518]

Telangiectasia

True telangiectases occur in the conjunctiva and reveal interesting patterns of vascular anomalies. Especially relevant are the dilatations of the conjunctival vessels which occur with the several systemic telangiectases. These include the syndrome of ataxia-telangiectasia (Louis-Barr syndrome),[524] ceramide trihexosidase deficiency (Fabry's disease),[361, 397, 536, 674] hereditary telangiectasia (Rendu-Osler disease),[574, 690] and trigeminal hemangiomatosis (Sturge-Weber syndrome; Fig. 6).

Despite the common denominator—telangiectasia—in all these entities the conjunctival manifestation is more that of a nonspecific dilatation of vessels and would not in itself warrant the designation of telangiectasis. Perhaps this is the reason that so many patients with these entities give the history of having had prolonged treatment for a supposed "conjunctivitis."

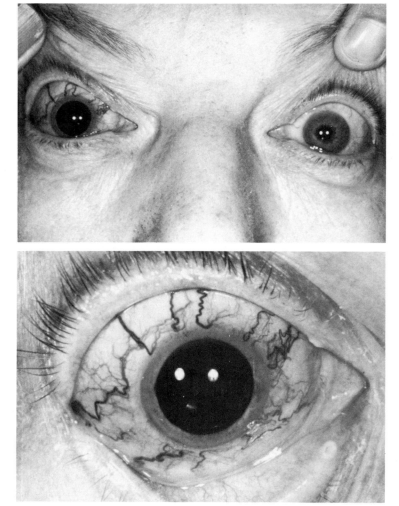

Figure 4   Unilateral exophthalmus and congestion in a patient with a shunt between dural vessels and cavernous sinus. (The pupillary mydriasis is artifactual.)

*The patient was a 69 year old woman who had developed the ocular signs sponta-
neously five months previously. Diagnosis was made by arteriography.*

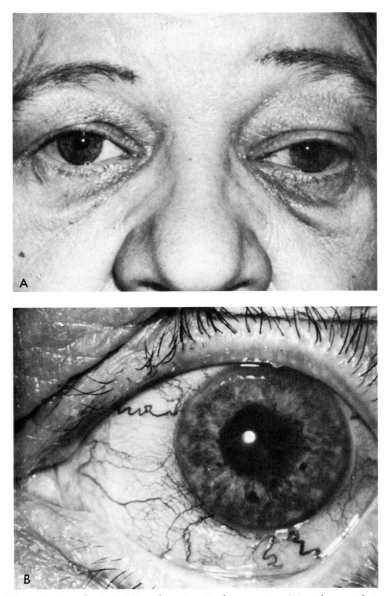

Figure 5 Pseudoptosis (A) and conjunctival congestion (B) with carotid stenosis.

The patient was a 57 year old woman with complete stenosis of the left internal carotid artery. Arteriography demonstrated flow by way of the external carotid artery and thence retrograde flow in the ophthalmic artery into the circle of Willis.

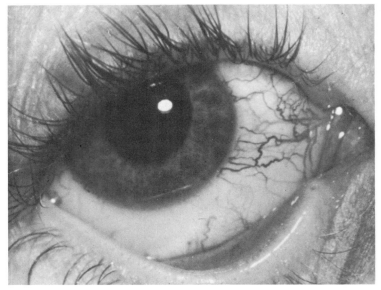

Figure 6   Dilatation of conjunctival vessels in ataxia-telangiectasia.

The patient was an 11 year old girl with the classic syndrome of telangiectasia of skin and eyes with progressive ataxia.

SLUDGING

Slowing of the circulation with consequently abnormal clumping of the red cells is called blood sludging[392] and is especially evident by slit-lamp biomicroscopy of the conjunctiva. The separation of red cells from plasma ("cattle-trucking") which is normally visible in conjunctival capillaries[380] becomes, with sludging, conspicuous in the veins as well, and occasionally in arteries.

Blood sludging occurs in any condition with increased viscosity or retarded circulation[317, 679] and may be the starting point for thrombosis.[638] It has been observed in polycythemia, multiple myeloma, and Waldenström's macroglobulinemia[78, 495] and is reversed by plasmaphoresis (Fig. 7).[440] Sludging occurring with sickle cell disease is said to increase at the times of sickle cell crises.[289] It occurs with cryoglobulinemia[164, 517] and may then be enhanced by local cooling of the conjunctiva. Some observers have claimed that sludging is seen with hypertension,[420] migraine,[58a] coronary sclerosis,[678] and simply with age.[215, 380] It may be induced by hypothermia (during anesthesia)[380, 401a] and experimentally in animals by either slowing the circulation or increasing the viscosity of the blood.[494] Some degree of sludging is said to become evident whenever the sedimentation rate exceeds 30 mm.[317]

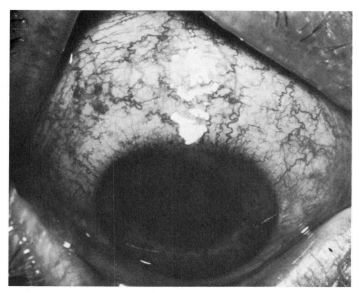

Figure 7 Stasis of conjunctival vessels with polycythemia.

The patient was a 43 year old man with prominent conjunctival vessels as part of his polycythemia. He had been treated for a presumed conjunctivitis.

CHEMOSIS

Chemosis is simply edema of the conjunctiva. It has a special name because it has a special appearance; this is due to the extraordinary looseness of the conjunctiva and the leakiness of conjunctival vessels. Although some degree of edema accompanies all inflammatory and congestive processes, the term chemosis is usually reserved for those cases in which the edema is disproportionately greater than would be expected from the vascular reaction (Fig. 8).

Chemosis of the conjunctiva is characterized by a pillowlike swelling of the conjunctiva which, in severe cases, protrudes between the lids in a grotesque and frightening fashion. Its color varies from a lemon yellow in mild cases to a fiery red in severe cases. It may result from vascular hypoosmolality but it is then usually of mild degree. More severe chemosis results from allergic states or from orbital stasis and, perhaps most commonly, with congestive dysthyroid exophthalmos.

HEMORRHAGE

The conjunctiva affords a unique opportunity to study gross and petechial hemorrhages not only because of its unique accessibility but

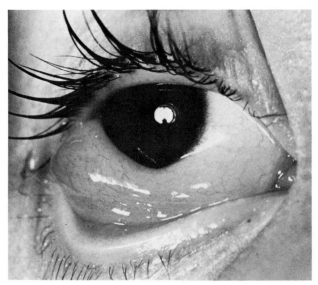

Figure 8   Chemosis.

The patient was a four year old girl who developed severe itching of the lids and edema of the conjunctiva, believed to be on an allergic basis.

also because patients are generally alarmed by the sudden red spots on their eyes and seek consultation whereas they would tend to ignore similar spots elsewhere.

Gross hemorrhages involving much or all of the conjunctiva occur commonly in middle-aged or older persons without apparent cause (Fig. 9). They often occur at night and are first observed, since they cause no symptoms, only when the patient looks in the mirror. They occur idiopathically and although occasionally associated with hemorrhagic diatheses[375, 521] they are not usually associated with hypertension or arteriosclerosis. Despite their alarming appearance, they absorb without sequelae.

On the other hand, gross ecchymoses of the lids, often associated with conjunctival hemorrhage, point to deep-seated orbital disease and suggest trauma, neoplasm, or a hemorrhagic diathesis.

In contrast to gross hemorrhage, petechiae of the bulbar or palpebral conjunctiva occur with various local and systemic diseases and often reflect an abnormal capillary fragility.[538] Splinter hemorrhages may appear with any febrile illness or blood dyscrasia but are especially noteworthy in subacute bacterial endocarditis, having the same significance as splinter hemorrhages beneath the fingernails (Fig. 10). They also occur with various forms of purpura and at one time were said to have been frequent in vitamin C deficient states. With trichin-

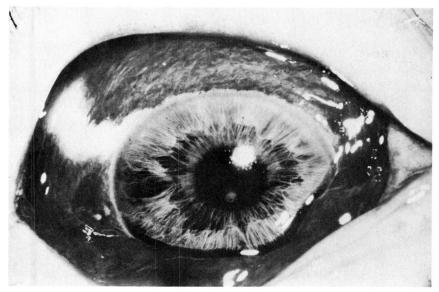

Figure 9 Massive conjunctival hemorrhage.

The patient was a 76 year old woman who developed the conjunctival hemorrhage without apparent cause and without pain or other subjective symptoms.

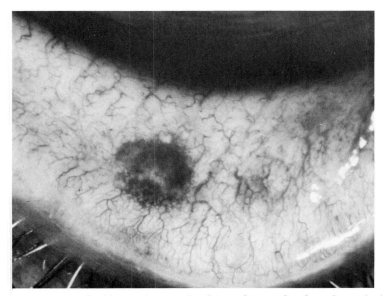

Figure 10 Petechial hemorrhage with subacute bacterial endocarditis. The lower lid has been everted to expose the palpebral conjunctiva.

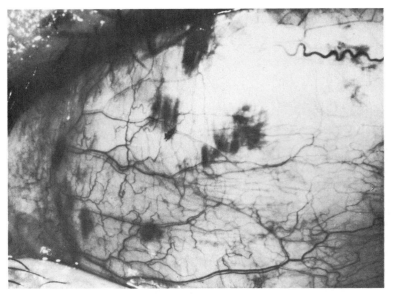

Figure 11   Multiple conjunctival hemorrhages with menses.

The patient was a 20 year old girl who had had several episodes of spontaneous hemorrhage with her menses.

osis the conjunctival hemorrhages accompany marked swelling of the lids and painful ophthalmoplegia. Rare instances have been noted with migraine and with the menstrual cycle (Fig. 11).[304]

MORPHOLOGIC CHANGES IN CONJUNCTIVAL VESSELS

Local dilatations, saccular outpouchings and microaneurysms of the conjunctival vessels have been ascribed to various systemic vasculopathies (Fig. 12). Some observers have described characteristic dilatations of the vessels in diabetes thought to be analogous to the microaneurysms of diabetic retinopathy.[152, 231, 287] Others have failed to demonstrate significant changes[88] while still others have reported them as transient abnormalities unrelated to the retinopathy or to the control of diabetes.[419] Cumulative evidence at present suggests that although dilatation and tortuosities of the conjunctival vessels may be statistically more frequent in diabetes, they are not morphologically distinctive[8] and have no significant relationship to the retinal microaneurysms.[4, 418] To emphasize this difference, some authors suggest that the vascular changes be called "micropools"[138] or simply "capillary dilatations"[233] rather than microaneurysms.

Similar changes in the conjunctival vessels have been described with hypertension and arteriosclerosis and have been claimed to reflect the state of the microvasculature in the heart[139, 178, 304] and in the

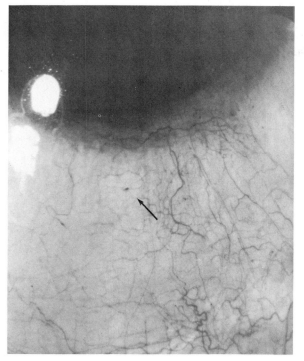

Figure 12 Saccular dilatation of conjunctival vessel (indicated by arrow).
The patient was a 44 year old man who had no known systemic disease.

brain.[177] One observer reported that ingestion of a fatty meal caused sludging and stasis in the conjunctival vessels of coronary-prone persons to a much greater extent than of normal persons.[227] These observations merit confirmation and controlled study.

The most exhaustive analysis of the conjunctival circulation has been carried out in the sickle cell hemoglobinopathies.[201, 233, 242, 262, 289, 392, 430, 506, 507] While some of the changes are nonspecific, a comma-shaped dilatation has been thought to be pathognomonic of sickle cell disease,[506] being found in the majority of patients with SS disease, inconstantly with SC disease, and absent in those with normal hemoglobins.[117] These dilatations are associated with stagnation of the blood in the adjacent lumen and have their histologic basis in swelling of the endothelium.[233]

ARCUS SENILIS AND JUVENILIS

Arcus senilis is the common white ring at the periphery of the cornea in middle-aged or older persons (Fig. 13). It is popularly believed

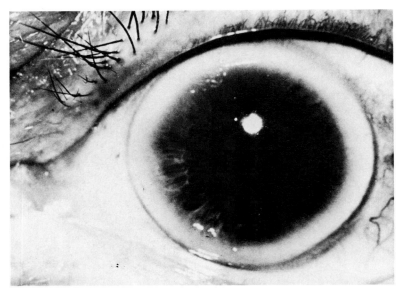

Figure 13 Arcus senilis. Characteristic is the white ring encircling the cornea but separated from the limbus by a narrow clear interval.

The patient was a 75 year old man whose blood cholesterol level was 365 mg per 100 ml. Medical examination disclosed no overt evidence of cardiac or vascular disease.

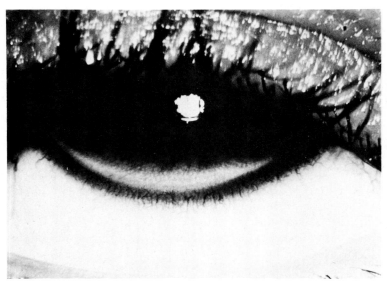

Figure 14 Arcus juvenilis, xanthelasma of the lids, and tendinous xanthomas of the knees in a patient with familial hypercholesteremia.

The patient was a 10 year old girl with a serum cholesterol level of 665 mg per 100 ml. Several other members of the family had a similar syndrome.

(Illustration continued on opposite page.)

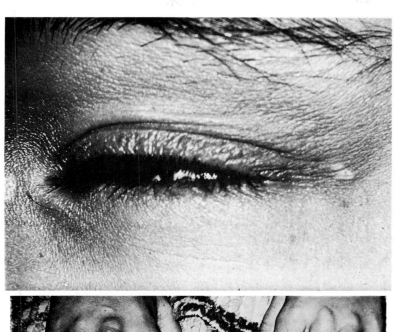

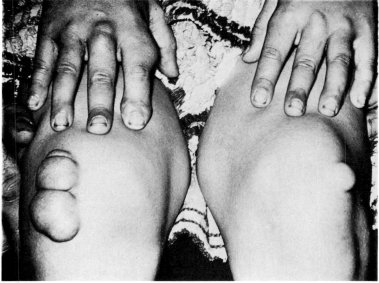

Figure 14 Continued.

to indicate atherosclerosis in the rest of the body. This arcus does represent lipid infiltration from the blood and is not a degenerative phenomenon.[106] However, the similarity to atherosclerosis goes no further. If one discounts the factor of age alone and excludes certain familial hypercholesterolemias, there is no convincing correlation of the ordinary arcus senilis with coronary occlusion nor with other systemic vascular disease.[347]

On the other hand, a similar arcus occurring at a young age, the arcus juvenilis, may be associated significantly with hypercholesteremia and, together with xanthelasma of the eyelids and tendinous xanthomas elsewhere, constitutes a clinical triad (Fig. 14).

These patients, in whom the hypercholesteremia is usually familial and in whom the serum level exceeds 400 mg per 100 ml, *do* have a high incidence of atherosclerosis and the arcus in them *does* correlate with coronary occlusion. These patients represent Types II and III hyperbetalipoproteinemia[217, 547] in which cholesterol is elevated with or without concomitant hypertriglyceridemia.

A lipid arcus can be produced in rabbits by feeding cholesterol. This is widely assumed to be the experimental counterpart of the arcus in man since these animals also develop fatal atherosclerosis. The level of cholesterolemia in rabbits, however, is greatly in excess of that in man and the histopathology in rabbits consists primarily of a cellular reaction to the lipid overloading rather than to acellular inundation of the tissue as occurs in the human arcus. A further point of difference is the conspicuous neovascularization of the rabbit arcus whereas this is characteristically absent in the human case.

Contrary to general opinion, therefore, the rabbit model does not provide a facsimile of the arcus in man.

SUMMARY

The outer part of the eye often reveals evidence of systemic vascular disease. Jaundice, anemia, bleeding tendencies, excessive metallic ions in the blood, and lipemia present characteristic appearances in the conjunctiva and episclera.

Slit-lamp biomicroscopy permits detection of blood sludging in hyperviscosity syndromes, crystalline deposits in cystinosis (sometimes in dysproteinemia), and calcium deposits in hypercalcemia and hyperphosphatemia.

Congestion of the conjunctival vessels, commonly seen with conjunctivitis, occurs passively with increased venous stasis and actively with alterations in arterial flow. The appearance of congestion may also result from conjunctival telangiectasia. However, the type of congestion is distinctly different in each of these.

Sludging or stasis of blood is seen with hyperviscosity syndromes and with conditions that slow the circulation. It is best appreciated by slit-lamp biomicroscopy.

The looseness of conjunctival tissue makes it vulnerable to profuse edema (chemosis) or to hemorrhage. Both conditions are usually benign and reversible. However, conjunctival hemorrhage associated with ecchymoses in the lids may indicate deep-seated abnormalities, and isolated hemorrhages in the conjunctiva may reflect subacute bacterial endocarditis, trichinosis, or bleeding diatheses.

Characteristic morphologic changes in the conjunctival vessels have been reported in diabetes, sickle cell hemoglobinopathy, and several other vasculopathic abnormalities. The considerable variation in normal conjunctival patterns makes the evaluation of these changes difficult.

Arcus senilis shows, in general, poor correlation with coronary and arteriosclerotic disease, except insofar as both increase with age, but the arcus juvenilis with familial hypercholesterolemia is significantly associated with atheromatous disease.

CHAPTER 2

FUNDUS

NORMAL FUNDUS AND VARIATION WITH AGE

The three cardinal features of the normal fundus relate to the disc (or papilla), the retinal vessels, and the general background (Fig. 15).

The disc is, of course, the exit channel for the nerve fibers from the retina and the site of incoming and outgoing vessels to and from the retina. Since one is accustomed to viewing the disc with the 15-fold magnification of the direct ophthalmoscope, it may come as a surprise to learn that the disc diameter is only 1.0 to 1.5 mm. For op-

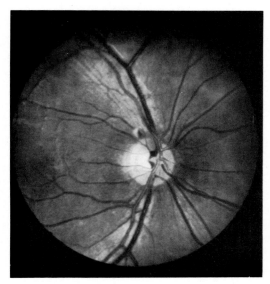

Figure 15 Normal fundus in an 18 year old man.

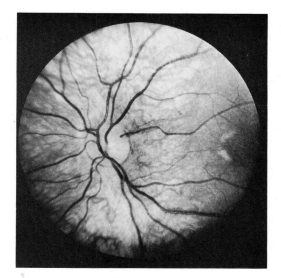

Figure 16 Normal blond fundus revealing the pattern of the choroidal vessels (and incidentally a cilioretinal artery).

tical reasons it appears relatively small in the hyperopic eye and large in the myopic eye.

The disc is pink on the nasal side and pinkish white on the temporal side. This color, imparted by the superimposed papillary capillaries, changes to all white with optic atrophy. The temporal edges are sharp and flat, although often accompanied by pigmented margins, while the nasal edges are relatively blurred and elevated. With hyperopia the entire circumference may become indistinct and simulate papilledema.

A funnel-shaped depression, the physiologic cup, usually occupies the center of the disc. This cup may vary in size without significance but in glaucoma its margin approaches the edge of the disc and threatens the integrity of the nerve fibers.

The vessels on the nerve head comprise the central artery and vein together with their branches. The artery is a direct branch of the ophthalmic artery and subdivides at the level of the disc, or close to it, into four main branches, one for each quadrant of the eye. In approximately one quarter of all cases, one or more cilioretinal arteries derived from the choroid enter the temporal edge of the disc and supply an area of the retina between the papilla and macula (Fig. 16).

The central retinal vein exits through the center of the disc and drains into the venous plexus of the orbit. Occasionally a retinochoroidal vein, analogous to the cilioretinal artery but less common, drains blood from part of the temporal retina into the choroid.

Estimation of the diameters of the retinal arteries may be accomplished by direct measurement or through fundus photography[126, 159, 160, 319, 486] but these methods are fraught with artifacts and do not provide the important panorama that is available by simple ophthalmoscopy.

The major arteries and veins are easily distinguishable. The arteries are smaller, brighter red, and run a straighter course than the veins. They usually lie superficial in the retina and anterior to the veins at the arteriovenous (AV) crossings. In young persons the arteries cross the veins at obtuse angles but with advancing age they develop a right angulation and frequently an obvious compression of the veins (see p. 44).

The finer vascular pattern is obscured ophthalmoscopically by the orange background of the choroid, but histologic mounts reveal an impressively regular alternation of the terminal arterioles and venules.

What are called retinal vessels are, of course, the blood columns within the vessels. With the exception of the parapapillary regions, the walls are normally transparent and become visible only under pathologic circumstances.

The retinal artery shows no expansile pulsation under normal conditions, for the retinal diastolic pressure is well above the intraocular pressure, but the retinal vein commonly pulsates at its exit from the disc, that is, at the site of lowest venous pressure. This pulsation reflects changes in the *intraocular* pressure with each cardiac beat rather than a change in the venous pressure. The vein collapses as the pressure within the eye exceeds that within the vein. The presence of venous pulsation has no clinical significance except that it rules out increased intracranial pressure in questionable cases of papilledema.[670] Spontaneous pulsation of the artery, on the other hand, is always of pathologic significance, indicating an abnormally low retinal diastolic pressure or high (glaucomatous) intraocular pressure.

The fundus background varies from a bright orange color in blond individuals to a chocolate brown in the Negro. The variation is due to the amounts of melanin in the choroid and pigment epithelium. The maze of choroidal vessels is visible in lightly complected persons (Fig. 16) but it may be seen only in those dark complected persons who have lost much of the pigment of the pigment epithelium. This attrition of pigment occurs regularly with age so that the fundi of older persons assume a tessellated appearance, with vessels and interstitial pigment of the choroid forming a characteristic mosaic.

Highlights reflected from the surface of the retina are prominent in young persons and may confuse observers unaccustomed to ophthalmoscopy. They are the brilliant lights that move with the changing positions of the ophthalmoscope and often delineate irregularities of the internal limiting membrane caused by the underlying nerve fibers and vessels. In the third or fourth decade of life they become inconspicuous or absent.

The central fundus warrants special comment. It is normally darker over a wide central area but presents at the posterior pole a single punctate highlight that moves parallactically in a direction opposite to that of the ophthalmoscope. This reflex derives from the foveal concavity and indicates an intact inner surface of this important part of the retina. The choroid behind the macula is thicker and contains more plentiful vessels, thereby imparting a diffuse redness to this central area and obscuring the individual vessels. The individual choroidal vessels are consequently more visible toward the periphery.

METHODS OF EXAMINATION

Ophthalmoscopy

Study of the fundus oculi affords an aesthetically pleasing as well as clinically informative part of the physical examination. It should not be done casually.

A few words about ophthalmoscopes and ophthalmoscopy are in order. The usual instrument for examination of the fundus is the *direct* ophthalmoscope (Fig. 17). It contains a series of lenses of varying dioptric power that permit sequential focusing from the front to the back of the eye. It is best to start with a plus 4 or 5 diopter lens at several inches from the eye to determine the clarity of the pupil and to allow time for the patient to steady his gaze. Then, by decreasing the lens power and simultaneously moving closer to the eye the fundus comes into view. The disc situated 10 to 15 degrees to the nasal side of

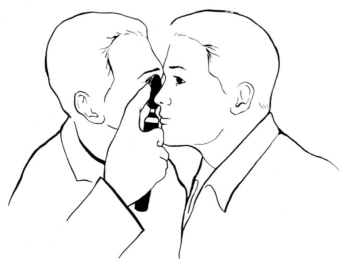

Figure 17   Direct ophthalmoscopy.

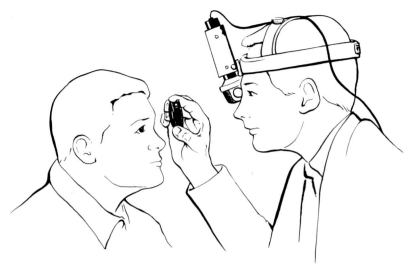

Figure 18   Indirect ophthalmoscopy. A lens is interposed between the examiner and patient.

the posterior pole is most satisfactory for focusing. This usually requires a minus 3 lens, with less power for examination of hyperopic eyes and more power for myopic eyes.

A more sophisticated method of examination is obtained by the *indirect* ophthalmoscope. The instruments in general use consist of a collimated light source strapped to the examiner's forehead and a focusing lens (usually plus 15 diopters) which the examiner holds between his own eyes and those of the patient (Fig. 18). The advantages of the indirect ophthalmoscope include: the larger field available for examination, the greater accessibility of the peripheral fundus, the greater penetrability of cloudy media with the bright light, and, most especially, the three dimensional visualization of the fundus. These advantages are desirable for ophthalmoscopy of uncooperative patients, of eyes with nystagmus, incipient cataracts, and cloudy vitreous, and of eyes with detached retinas or intraocular tumors in which elevated landmarks are important criteria. The disadvantages of indirect ophthalmoscopy are the inverted image of the fundus, the necessity of a dilated pupil, and, particularly, the considerable experience which the method requires for its execution. Those who have persevered have found it rewarding.

Biomicroscopy

Although biomicroscopy is used chiefly to examine anterior parts of the eye (Fig. 19), it may be adapted with either special lenses in front of, or contact lenses on, the eye to supplement examination of

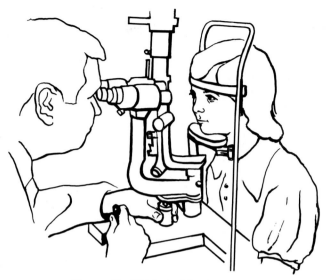

Figure 19 Slit-lamp biomicroscopy.

the fundus. It is especially useful for studying the relative depths of lesions in the retina and choroid but it requires considerable practice and is not recommended for general use.

Fluoroangiography

Since the early 1960s when fluoroangiography was introduced as a method for visualizing the vessels in the back of the eye,[443, 496] a large literature, including several atlases, has accumulated.[363, 552, 587, 680]

The customary technique for fluoroangiography consists of injecting 5 to 10 cc of 10 per cent fluorescein into the antecubital vein and then taking photographs of the fundus in rapid sequence so as to show the entrance and transmission of the fluorescein through the vessels.[196, 281] Two or more pictures are taken per second with special filters to eliminate extraneous light. Under favorable conditions the pictures illustrate the vascular patterns, including the capillary plexuses, and are comparable to the histologic preparations of flat mounts. In addition they provide information on the hemodynamics that would otherwise be impossible to obtain.

The fluorescein is essentially nontoxic. Thousands of tests have been performed with no more than transient nausea or mild allergic reactions.[623] However, transient loss of consciousness with bronchospasm[576] has been reported in one patient, respiratory distress in another (relieved by adrenalin),[422] and a single case of death concomitant with the injection.[568] Accordingly, those who undertake fluorescein angiography should have oxygen and adrenalin available for the rare emergency which might arise.

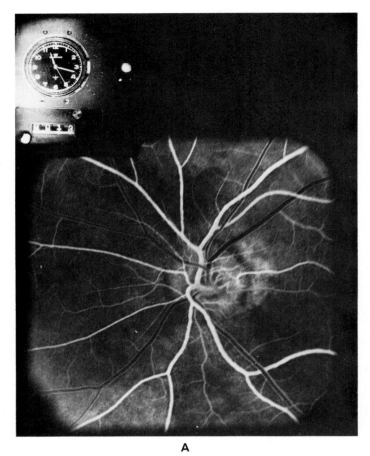

A

Figure 20 Normal fluoroangiograms of: *(A)* arterial phase with dye in the arteries, and

(*Illustration continued on opposite page.*)

Fluorescein* enters the eye in 8 to 12 seconds after beginning the injection. The entire fundus lights up as the fluorescein enters the choroid but the central fundus is darker owing to the greater amount of pigment in this area. As the choroid lights up, or soon thereafter (rarely before), fluorescein enters the retinal arteries and within 1 to 2 seconds it has passed into the veins (Fig. 20). A striking feature of this early venous phase is the lamination of the fluorescein in the larger veins.

A cilioretinal artery will light up with the choroidal filling and may therefore precede the fluorescence of the retinal vessels. For the same reason

---

*Actually the injected fluorescein promptly binds to serum albumen. In speaking of fluorescein transfer and leakage, therefore, one is referring to a protein-bound dye.

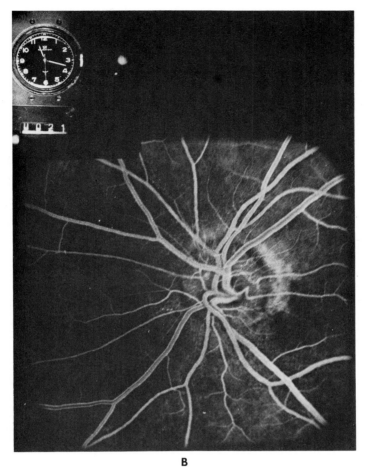

B

Figure 20 Continued. (B) venous phase with dye in arteries and veins (showing lamination in some).

the disc may also fluoresce before the retinal vessels since part of the papillary circulation comes from the choroid.

The fluorescence clears from the *retinal* vessels in 5 to 10 minutes, leaving a faint glow of protein-bound fluorescein in the blood stream. It does not normally leak out of the retinal vessels. By contrast, fluorescein normally leaks out of the *choroidal* vessels to form a luminous background of the choroid and nerve head that persists for an hour or more.

Recent cinefluoroangiography has been used to provide a more continuous record of the circulation[250] but this technique has a practical limit in the amount of light the patient will tolerate. Fluoroangiography by television[251] requires less light but sacrifices resolution.

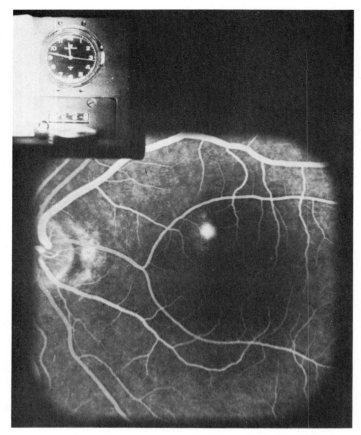

Figure 21   Demonstration of a leak by fluoroangiography.

The leak which in this patient was due to central serous retinopathy is evident by the fluorescent white spot above and nasal to the macula. It increased progressively over a period of several minutes and remained after the dye had left the vessels.

While fluoroangiograms reveal the normal vascular patterns impressively, their chief value is the detection of obstruction to flow, defects in the pigment epithelium, pathologic vessel formation, and, most especially, abnormal leaks from the choroidal and retinal blood vessels (Fig. 21). Retinal vascular anomalies are demonstrated most vividly.[551]

Visualization of the choroidal vessels by fluoroangiography is handicapped by filtration in the overlying pigment epithelium and choriocapillaris. However, new dyes (indocyanine) emitting longer wavelengths than fluorescein afford greater penetrability and may eventually be found useful.[318, 398, 410] Heretofore, the larger choroidal vessels have been visualized only in late fluoroangiograms as silhouettes against a fluorescent sclera.

Ophthalmodynamometry (Ocular Sphygmomanometry)

The blood pressure of the retinal arteries may be easily measured by raising the intraocular pressure through an external force applied to the sclera and simultaneously observing the arterial pulsation on the nerve head (Fig. 22). The first induced pulsation corresponds to the diastolic pressure while the eventual elimination of pulsation and maintained collapse of the artery corresponds to the systolic pressure. The popular instrument for applying the pressure is a spring-loaded plunger within a sliding barrel and is known as the Bailliart ophthalmodynamometer. The scale is calibrated in mm Hg and corresponds approximately to the intraocular pressure which in turn is exerted on the wall of the artery. More quantitative methods are possible[279, 491, 675] but usually are unnecessary since comparative measurements between the two eyes are the main criteria.

A local anesthetic is instilled on the eye, and the foot-plate of the dynamometer is placed on the sclera several millimeters behind the limbus. The end-point may be read off the scale by a second observer or may be stopped by a manual control at any point when the observer is unassisted. The measurements are facilitated by using indirect ophthalmoscopy with a dilated pupil but this requires a two-man team.

The diastolic end-points are easy to obtain and the pressure causes no appreciable discomfort to the patient. The arterial pulsation at these diastolic levels has a distinctly snapping quality that is unmistakable. The systolic end-point, however, is less sharp and causes some discomfort to the patient. Moreover, there is a danger of trauma from slippage of the foot-plate on the sclera or even of permanent occlusion of the central retinal artery.[572, 617] Unless especially indicated, therefore, systolic pressures are not obtained routinely.[323, 324, 617] In the absence of an ophthalmodynamometer, arterial pressures may be roughly estimated by manual pressure against the lid during ophthalmoscopy.

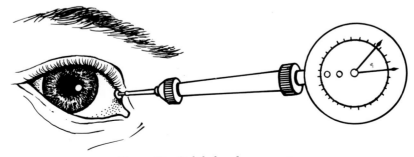

Figure 22   Ophthalmodynamometry.

The expansile (or collapsing) pulsation must be differentiated from the common transmitted pulsation which has little or no significance. The transmitted pulsation consists of slight lateral displacement of the artery without change in its caliber. It occurs most commonly in persons with high mean arterial pressures and is enhanced by unusual rigidity and tortuosity of the arteries.

The pressures are usually obtained with the patient in the sitting position but comparative measurements in the supine and standing position are occasionally indicated in cases of suspected postural hypotension.[607]

The pressure levels vary from person to person but are normally equal to within 15 per cent in the two eyes of any one person. They usually amount to from 50 to 75 per cent of the brachial pressures. What is actually determined is the pressure in the ophthalmic artery rather than that of the normal retinal artery since the act of arresting the circulation will automatically raise the pressure to that of the feeding vessel. The observed pressure in the retinal arteries is probably 14 to 17 mm higher than the normal pressure in the retinal artery.[648]

Retinal blood pressures have local significance in detecting retinal artery occlusions but their chief value is in evaluating carotid occlusive disease. A difference of arterial pressure greater than 20 per cent between the two eyes or significant difference in pulse pressures[502] suggests carotid stenosis. On the other hand, an equal pressure in the two eyes does not rule out carotid disease since collateral circulation from either the ipsilateral external carotid artery or the contralateral internal carotid may maintain normal ophthalmic artery pressures despite the carotid occlusion.[124, 324, 532, 562, 609, 611, 613, 617]

To test for collateral carotid circulation a compression test has been recommended.[475, 606, 629, 672] Neck pressure on the side of the occlusion will cause no effect on the retinal artery pressure whereas pressure on the side of the patent carotid artery will drop the arterial pressure in both eyes. This test may be indicated at times but is not without danger since it jeopardizes the entire carotid circulation to the brain.

Arterial pulsation occurs whenever the retinal diastolic pressure is less than the intraocular pressure; that is, when it is less than 20 mm Hg. It is thus encountered with aortic regurgitation, carotid stenosis, aortic arch disease, and vasomotor collapse. Spontaneous arterial pulsation may also occur in the presence of a normal arterial pressure when the intraocular pressure is sufficiently elevated (glaucoma).

Obstruction of the ophthalmic artery can usually be distinguished from that of the carotid by the quality of pulsation induced by ophthalmodynamometry. With ophthalmic artery obstruction, the pulsation is weak or absent. As diastole is approached, the artery simply collapses and then refills slowly as the external pressure is released. It does not have the snapping quality which is present normally and which may be present even with carotid stenosis.

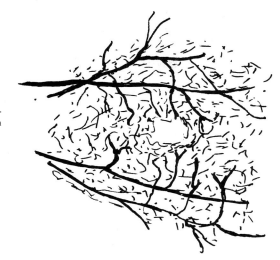

Purkinje pattern of the retinal vessels seen by trans-scleral illumination.

Endoscopy

Endoscopy is the procedure of visualizing structures and opacities in one's own eye. The larger blood vessels in the retina can be visualized subjectively by transilluminating the sclera in a darkened room. The observer looks to one extreme side while the assistant oscillates a bright small light focused on the sclera. The main retinal vessels, up to the second or third order of branches, stand out in silhouette against a luminous background (Fig. 23). This is called the Purkinje pattern and has some clinical usefulness in eyes with opaque media. Perception of the Purkinje pattern means that the retina is in place. It is, however, too coarse a test and the images are too evanescently seen to permit detailed analysis of the vessels.

The macular capillaries can be seen endoscopically by gazing at some uniformly luminous background (such as the clear blue sky) and

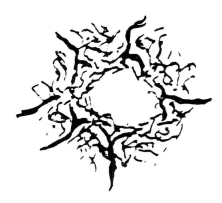

Figure 24   Pattern of macular capillaries seen by endoscopy.

oscillating a pin-hole aperture in front of one's eye. With a little pa-
tience one can visualize the capillary network about the macula and
the avascular central "hole" of the fovea (Fig. 24). The clinical significance of this method has not been explored sufficiently to permit an
authoritative opinion of its potential usefulness but it has not so far
revealed any obvious pathology.

Electroretinography, Electro-oculography and Evoked Cortical Potentials

Although practicable only in centers for specialized services,
these electrical tests can provide important information on retinal
function.

The electroretinogram (ERG) depends on a transient millivoltage
change in the electrical potential between the cornea and retina in
response to a flash of light (Fig. 25). Its presence indicates that the
photoreceptive layer of the retina is intact but gives no indication of
the status of the inner retinal layers. Thus it may be normal despite
loss of the entire inner portions of the retina from central retinal artery
occlusion but will be weak or absent with choroidal vasculopathies or
degenerations that destroy the outer portion of the retina. It is not a
sensitive test; extensive portions of the outer layers must be lost
before reliable changes in the electroretinogram can be detected.

The abundant literature on electroretinography deals chiefly with degenerative disease, especially retinitis pigmentosa and drug effects, rather than
with vasculopathies.

The electrooculogram (EOG) depends on stationary differences
in potential between retina and cornea[170] rather than on changes induced by light. It is usually measured by use of bitemporal or naso-
temporal electrodes which record changes in potential with horizontal
movements of the eye. The electro-oculogram has much the same sig-

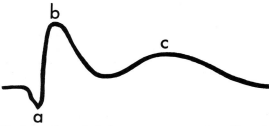

Figure 25   The form of a typical electroretinogram induced by a flash of light. The
graph indicates a change in potential between cornea and retina. The *a* wave is a negative deflection arising in the photoreceptors or outer layer of the retina. The *b* wave is a
positive deflection arising largely in the glial (Müller) cells of the middle retinal layers
and the *c* wave is believed to reflect a potential change in the pigment epithelium of the
retina.

nificance as the electroretinogram and is particularly useful in degenerative diseases rather than in vasculopathies.[36] For obvious reasons,
it is especially adaptable for tracking eye movements.

Cortically evoked potentials are recorded by tapping off changes
in the occipital potentials that result from exposing the eye to flashes
of light. This method has been made possible by integrative techniques which select and summate the significant signals out of a noisy
background. It supplements the ERG and EOG methods in detecting
disease of the neural conduction system. Cortically evoked potentials
are unelicitable with loss of the inner retinal layers even though the
ERG and EOG are normal. It further supplements the ERG, which is
responsive to large areas of photoreceptor loss only, by being especially sensitive to loss of macular vision. This is due to the dispropor-
tionate contribution which macular vision makes to the electrical activity of the occiput.

Measurement of the visually evoked potentials is important for
evaluating visual functions, especially in the presence of opaque
media which prevent ordinary means of testing, but it has no special
relevance to vascular disease.

ANATOMO-PATHO-CLINICO CORRELATIONS

Retina

The retina is a composite membrane, 0.5 mm thick in the disc area
and considerably less than this in the periphery. It is anatomically attached to the rest of the eyeball only about the disc posteriorly and the
ora serrata anteriorly. That it remains in place as well as it does is due
to the gelatinous vitreous on its inner surface and a polysaccharide
coating that holds the rods and cones to the pigment epithelium on its
outer surface. The occasional detachment of the retina (really a separation) is evidence that these factors are not always adequate.

From outer to inner surfaces, following the course of the neural
impulses (Fig. 26), the retina consists of the following layers: the photoreceptors or rods and cones; the so-called external limiting membrane which in reality is formed by the terminal bars coapting the
photoreceptive cells and the glial processes; the outer nuclear layer
comprising cell bodies of the photoreceptors; the outer reticular layer
comprising the synaptic junctions of the photoreceptor cells with the
next order of neurons; the inner (but not innermost) layer of nuclei
representing the neuronal bipolar cells and the glial (Müller) cells as
well as a few other cell types (horizontal and amacrine cells); the
inner reticular layer containing the synapses for the bipolar cells with
their next neuronal relay; the ganglion cell layer; the layer of nerve
fibers which are the axones of the ganglion cells and extend out of the

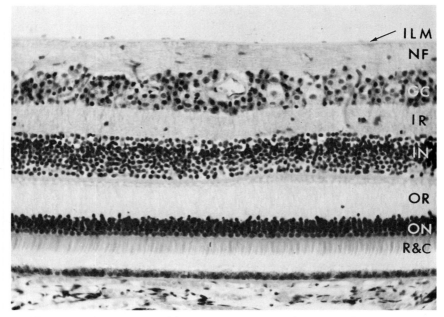

Figure 26 Cross-section of the retina near the macula. *R&C*, rods and cones; *ON*, outer nuclear layer; *OR*, outer reticular layer; *IN*, inner nuclear layer; *IR*, inner reticular layer; *GC*, ganglion cell layer; *NF*, nerve fiber layer; *ILM*, inner limiting membrane.

eye to form the optic nerves; and, finally, the internal limiting membrane or basement membrane of the Müller foot-plates.

The central area of the retina, designated the macula because of its yellow xanthophyll pigment, warrants special mention since it is anatomically adapted to provide maximal visual acuity (Fig. 27) and disturbances of it lead to disproportionately profound visual loss. The inner layers of the retina are attenuated in the center of the macula to form a concave depression called the fovea. Here the blood vessels are absent and the photoreceptors, which are almost entirely cones, are directly exposed to incoming light without the intermediary scattering that occurs elsewhere in the retina.

The outer reticular layer is modified in the macula to form radiating fibers, or Henle's fiber layer, that parallel the declivity of the fovea. (It is because of this radiating pattern that exudates, and sometimes hemorrhages, in the central area form a star-shaped figure.) About the fovea the ganglion cells are unusually abundant, supplying the foveal cones with a one-to-one connection with the brain and thereby enabling maximal visual resolution.

The blood vessels of the retina are confined to the innermost layers. The major arteries and veins course in the most superficial layers and are interconnected by hammock-like capillary plexuses that extend no deeper than the bipolar cell layer.

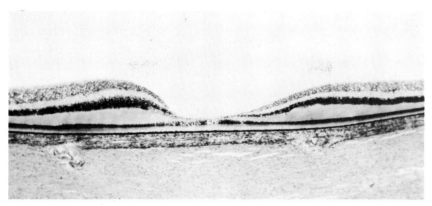

Figure 27 Cross-section at the posterior pole of the eye including the macular and paramacular regions of the retina. Noteworthy is the attenuation of all the retinal layers, except the photoreceptors, in the center of the macula.

The glia of the retina, called Müller's cells or Müller's fibers, not only provide physical support in the traditional sense but also serve metabolic functions that are ancillary to the circulation.[414] The blood vessels are everywhere ensheathed by these glia with no appreciable tissue space. Neurones obtain their vascular requirements only through the intermediary of these glial cells which have a special capacity for synthesis and storage of glycogen.[346]

The inner layers of the retina depend entirely on the retinal vascular system. Occlusion of the retinal artery causes disappearance of all the inner layers down to the mid-zone of the bipolar layer. The outer layers of the retina, on the other hand, remain intact since they can be effectively supplied by the choroid.

Histologic preparation of the retinal vessel system as whole mounts,[221] either by injection[22, 471] or by trypsin digestion[413] techniques, illustrates how elaborate and yet systematic is the capillary system of the retina (Fig. 28). These mounts raise many questions about the normal and pathologic hemodynamics of the retina which are only partially answered. The trypsin digest technique has demonstrated a duality of the cell types constituting the cell wall that, if not unique, is unlike that of most capillaries in the body. The endothelial cells form a nonfenestrated inner lining, bound together by tight junctions, while another cell type, which the author has called mural cell[415] but which others prefer to call intramural pericytes,[29] is contained within the wall substance of the capillary (Fig. 29). These latter cells are probably muscular and probably regulate the distribution of blood flow throughout the capillary bed in some as yet ill-understood manner. They may be analogous to pericytes elsewhere but have not as yet been shown to be contractile.[225]

The mural cells (intramural pericytes), identified in trypsin digest mounts by their round nuclei and heavy nuclear staining (with hema-

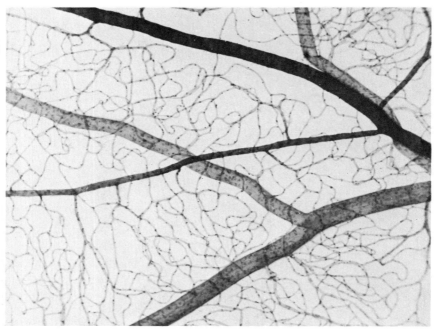

Figure 28   Sample of vessels from mid-periphery of retina prepared as flat mounts after trypsin digestion, illustrating the architecture of the microvasculature.

toxylin), and the endothelial cells, distinguished by their paler staining and ellipsoid nuclei, are normally distributed in approximately equal numbers throughout the capillaries. With ischemia the endothelial cells disappear first, leaving occluded capillaries with residual mural cells (Fig. 30).[545] These latter eventually disappear also, but the basement membrane remains indefinitely as a partially frayed scaffolding. This sequence of loss of endothelial cells, then of mural cells, occurs regularly in the retinal periphery, beginning in middle life and progressing to total occlusion of the vessels farthest from the arterial source.[416]

A further impelling reason for interest in these mural cells is that, while they seem to be more resistant to ischemia than are the endothelial cells, they are the primary target for diabetes. Substantial evidence indicates their selective disappearance accounts for the initial pathology in diabetic retinopathy (see p. 87).

The retinal capillaries have a uniform diameter of about 5μ; that is less than the diameter of the concave-convex red blood cells. High-speed cinephotography of the retinal circulation has shown streamlining of red blood cells with an exaggerated paraboloid deformation[225] similar to what has been shown in mesenteric capillaries where the change in shape was thought to facilitate exchange in gases with the extravascular tissue.[272]

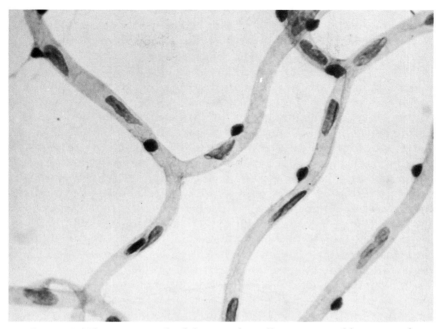

Figure 29 Photomicrograph of the retinal capillaries prepared by trypsin digestion illustrating the distinctive nuclei of the two cellular types of the retinal capillaries,
those of the mural cells and those of the endothelial cells.

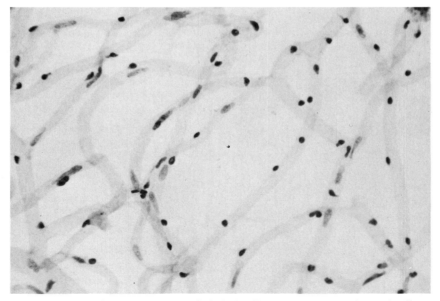

Figure 30 Relative paucity of endothelial cells in comparison with mural cells occurring in the mid-retinal periphery of a middle-aged person. This is a normal occurrence with either age or ischemia.

The basement membrane of the retinal capillaries consists of mucoprotein and collagen[151, 425] similar to that of vessels elsewhere but it is thicker than that of most capillaries and shows more obvious degenerative changes with age. These latter developments may be manifest in photomicroscopy by the sudanophilia of the walls and in electron microscopy by a Swiss cheese–like fenestration and thickening of the walls.

A remarkable feature of the retinal vasculature is the absence of neovasculogenesis within the retina in pathologic states. This contrasts with the lush proliferation of retina-derived vessels that have erupted into the vitreous. The abnormal vessels which are seen ophthalmoscopically in various conditions and often interpreted as new-formed vessels in the retina are found in flat mounts to be dilatations of antecedent capillaries. Vessels that grow into the vitreous, on the other hand, have characteristically large lumina with thin and leaky walls (see p. 55). Coming from the disc or the retina, they will form fronds in the vitreous or lie flat on the surface of the retina, depending on the integrity of the vitreous.

The nerve head consists chiefly of neural fibers (from the retina), astroglia, blood vessels to and from the retina, and a superficial capillary plexus that derives in part from the retinal vessels and a deep plexus from the peripapillary choroidal vessels (Fig. 31). These capillaries give the normally pink color to the disc, and their loss results in the pallor of optic atrophy.

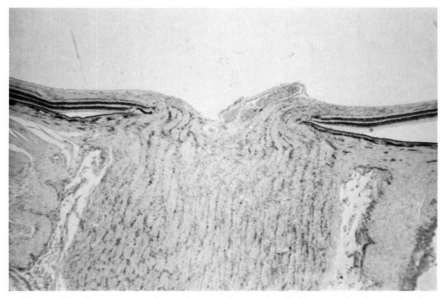

Figure 31 Cross-section through normal nerve head. (See text for description.)

The superficial plexuses on and adjacent to the disc have been called the radial peripapillary capillaries[470] and supply the nerve fibers to the disc. In contrast to other portions of the retina, the peripapillary capillaries run a relatively straight course with few anastomoses and end abruptly, abutting against the larger retinal arteries.[309, 643] These capillaries selectively atrophy (that is, lose their cellularity) with optic atrophy[97] including the atrophy caused by glaucoma.[308, 404, 689]

The central vessels on the disc differ from those in the retina in having better developed adventitia, muscular coat, and internal elastic lamina and in being susceptible to atheroma formation. The papillary retinal vessels thus represent the transition from artery to arteriole and correspond to similar transition in cerebral vessels of 100 to 200 μ in diameter.

An important anastomosis between the retinal and choroidal circulation occurs on the nerve head.[297] This becomes especially prominent with pathologic obstruction of the central vein at the lamina cribrosa with consequent distension of the bypass vessels on and about the disc.[385, 688]

One further anatomic feature that warrants mention is the fibrous sievelike structure, the lamina cribrosa, through which the nerve fibers and blood vessels exit from the eye. This presents a relatively rigid constraint preventing expansion of the vessels. It thus favors lodgment of calcific emboli in the artery and obstruction of the vein in the various hyperviscosity syndromes. Moreover, the central artery and vein are frequently bound together by a common adventitia during their transit through the lamina so that sclerotic changes in the arterial wall will cause secondary occlusion of the vein. The lamina cribrosa thus contributes importantly to the pathogenesis of retinal vascular accidents.

Choroid

Situated external to the retina and separated from it by the layer of pigment epithelial cells and by Bruch's hyaline membrane, the choroid lies internal to the sclera (Fig. 32). During life it is probably about 0.33 mm thick at the posterior pole and progressively thinner toward the periphery. Its chief constituents are blood vessels and pigment cells. The arterial supply enters the choroid posteriorly by a series of short ciliary arteries that penetrate the sclera about the optic nerve. The peripheral choroid is also supplied by recurrent branches of the major arterial circle in the ciliary body. The watershed area between these two systems is the common site for ischemic choroidal changes in the fundus periphery (see Elschnig spots, p. 80). The major venous drainage of the choroid is by way of the four vortex

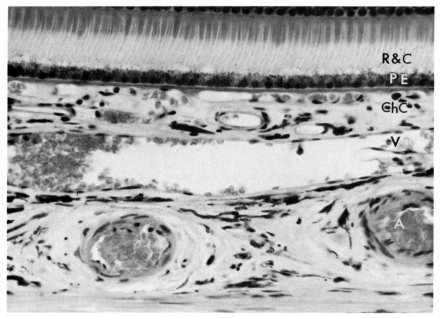

Figure 32 Cross-section of choroid, pigment epithelium, and photoreceptors. *R&C*, rods and cones; *PE*, pigment epithelium; *ChC*, choriocapillaris; *V*, vein; *A*, artery.

veins, one in each quadrant, that exit through the sclera halfway between the equator of the eye and the posterior pole.

So vascular is the choroid and so capable of varying its blood volume that some consider it erectile tissue. The arteries are situated predominately in the outermost part of the choroid while the veins occupy its bulk. The important capillary system of the choroid comprises a flat layer of sinusoids called the choriocapillaris situated just posterior to Bruch's membrane. One component of this membrane is the anterior wall of the choriocapillary sinuses; a rupture of Bruch's membrane is, therefore, a common cause of subretinal hemorrhage.

The choroidal arteries differ strikingly from the retinal arteries, a contrast which is of special interest since both are subjected to the same tissue pressure and arranged in a flat sheet of approximately equal dimensions. But whereas the retinal arteries have no elastica and only a diminutive muscularis (and are therefore really arterioles) the choroidal arteries have a substantial elastica and thick muscularis, signifying considerable control of the circulation at the local level. Further evidence of this autoregulation is the presence of mast cells which are normally present in the interstices of the choroid.

The choriocapillaris supplies the photoreceptors and outer layers of the retina through diffusion and processing in the pigment epithelium. It also acts undoubtedly as a cooling system for the focused visible and infrared energy absorbed in the pigment epithelium. As might be expected, the choriocapillaris, along with the rest of the choroid, is best developed beneath the macular area.

The endothelium lining the anterior wall of the choriocapillaris has fenestrations that, in contrast to the lining of retinal capillaries, is freely permeable to most blood constituents. The choroidal veins, also contrasting with those of the retina, react to inflammation by free outpouring of cells and serum into the adjacent tissue.

The arteries of the choroid are capable of atheromatosis and nodular hyalinization of their walls but the rich anastomoses, at least in the posterior regions of the eye, prevent the usual manifestations of ischemia.[702] In the periphery, however, the sparser choroidal vessels render the occlusive changes more devastating and account, undoubtedly, for the frequent focal or "pavement" degenerations and for the common loss of photoreceptors that occur regularly in eyes of elderly persons.

Overview

It is apparent from the foregoing sketches that the eye contains two vascular beds that are anatomically and functionally quite distinct.[10] What are called retinal arteries are really arterioles with only a diminutive muscularis, a negligible adventitia, and no elastic lamina. They are end arteries with strict territorial limitations that permit only a limited interarterial connection by way of the capillary bed. Moreover, these retinal vessels appear to be impermeable to all blood constituents except possibly oxygen and carbon dioxide.

The choroidal vasculature consists, by contrast, of arteries with thickly muscular walls, a substantial adventitia, and an appreciable internal elastic lamina. They possess some measure of autoregulation to extravascular pressure changes. The choroidal vessels have a rich overlap of territories with free connection through the choriocapillary sinusoids. The claim for arteriovenous shunts[434] is disputed.[25, 320, 701] The choriocapillaris and choroidal veins are freely permeable, permitting exudation and infiltration into the choroid.

Perhaps no other place in the body presents such a contrast in two vascular systems that are subjected to the same tissue pressure and derived from the same source.

SUMMARY

Especially noteworthy in the normal fundus is the color and sharpness of the disc, the distinction of arteries and veins, and the contribution of the choroid and pigment epithelium to the background appearance. The fundus is customarily viewed by direct ophthalmoscopy. More sophisticated methods of fundoscopy with their own advantages and disadvantages are indirect ophthalmoscopy, biomicroscopy, and fluoroangiography.

Other means of examining the eye include the following: ophthalmodynamometry for determining the blood pressure in the retinal artery, endoscopy for visualizing one's own vessels, electroretinography that records a change in corneoretinal potential in response to a flash of light or electrooculography that records the change in response to movements of the eye (both reflecting the integrity of the photoreceptive layer of the retina), and evoked cortical potentials that give some measure of macular function.

The retina comprises a complex membrane with three nuclear layers and two synaptic layers on which considerable processing of the visual impulses takes place. The macula is the central area in which the layers are attenuated to minimize scattering of the incoming light rays.

The retinal circulation provides the blood supply to the innermost layers and the choroidal circulation to the outermost avascular layers. The retinal vessels are best visualized as flat mounts prepared by trypsin digestion. Especially noteworthy is the thick and relatively impermeable wall of the capillaries with duplex cell type consisting of endothelium and mural cell.

The optic nerve comprises axones of the retinal ganglion cells, and the optic disc or papilla is the site of exit of these nerve fibers from the globe as they pass through the fenestrated portions of the sclera. The pinkness of the disc depends on capillaries derived from both the retinal and choroidal circulation. The disappearance of these capillaries produces the pallor of optic atrophy.

The choroid is a highly vascular membrane that supplies the photoreceptive layer of the retina and acts as a heat radiator or cooling system for light focused on the back of the eye. In contrast to the retinal circulation, it contains abundant anastomoses through its choriocapillary layer, and possesses a considerable capacity for autoregulation. Also in contrast to the retina its vessels are freely permeable to serum and formed elements of the blood.

Whereas the retinal arteries have no elastica and only a diminutive muscular coat and therefore do not show the pathologic changes of atherosclerosis, the choroidal arteries have substantial elastic and muscular constituents and therefore show pathologic changes comparable to larger arteries in the body.

CHAPTER 3

SIGNIFICANCE OF FUNDUS SIGNS

Narrowing and Tortuosity of Arteries

Evaluation of mild narrowing of the retinal arteries is rendered difficult by anatomic variations and by the refractive status of the eye. Thus, multiple branching will result in a small caliber of any one vessel; the vessels will *appear* to be small in hyperopia or large in myopia owing to the optical properties of ophthalmoscopy. It is better, therefore, to estimate the arterial diameter as a function of other landmarks in the fundus. This is ordinarily two thirds the size of the corresponding vein and maximally one tenth the diameter of the disc.

Notwithstanding these limitations, pathologic narrowing of the retinal arteries is usually obvious when it is moderate or severe. It is a valuable criterion in hypertension (see Chap. 5) in which both diffuse narrowing and focal constrictions occur. It is also characteristic of arterial occlusions, some cases of retinal atrophy, and is especially severe in the abiotrophies, such as retinitis pigmentosa, in which the photoreceptors have degenerated.

This paradoxic narrowing of the retinal arteries with degeneration of those portions of the retina not normally supplied by the retinal artery has been attributed to the higher oxygen availability resulting from the closer apposition of the retina to the inner retinal layers.[492]

Narrowing of the retinal arteries also occurs with excess oxygen[216, 593] (causing microinfarcts experimentally)[451] and may lead to a devastating occlusion in premature infants exposed to high oxygen atmospheres (see Retrolental Fibroplasia, p. 117). Yet hyperbaric oxygen has little effect on the retinal vessels of adults.[567]

Tortuosity of the retinal arteries increases with age and is often interpreted as a cognate sign of retinal arteriosclerosis (see Chap. 5). It may also occur congenitally with coarctation of the aorta and with congenital heart disease.

Congestion and Tortuosity of Veins

The retinal veins are one half again as wide as the corresponding arteries. With congestion they may exceed this difference several fold (Fig. 33). The blood then appears darker, in part because of the greater thickness of the veins and in part because of the greater proportion of unsaturated hemoglobin in the congested veins.

Important ancillary signs of retinal venous congestion are tortuosity of the venules, accentuation of the arteriovenous crossing phenomena, and occasionally microaneurysms.

The retinal veins may be dilated and tortuous congenitally but are especially dilated in hyperviscosity syndromes and in some cases of diabetes (see p. 130). They then often have a beaded or sausage-like configuration (Fig. 34). They are also distended with arterial occlusion,[298, 370] with congenital heart disease,[523] and with the excessive intraocular pressure of glaucoma, but the most extreme distension occurs, along with hemorrhagic retinopathy, in occlusion of the central retinal vein. Tributary occlusion causes less distension because of the collateral circulation.

Tortuosity of the veins is a feature of congenital arteriovenous shunts (Fig. 35), Fabry's disease, and several telangiectatic and vascular occlusive syndromes such as Leber's miliary aneurysms, Coats' disease, and Eales' disease (see p. 116). Although these are purely local vascular abnormalities in the eye they are frequently associated with alterations in the immunoglobulins.[219, 358, 365]

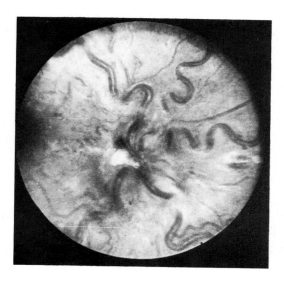

Figure 33 Severe congestion of retinal veins occurring in a patient with leukemia.

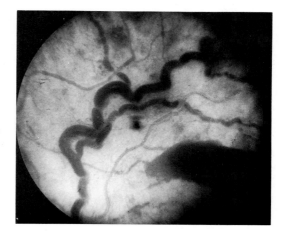

Figure 34 Sausage-like dilatation of vein and hemorrhagic retinopathy with macroglobulinemia. The Ostwald viscometer indicated a viscosity of 14 at 37°C.

Ensheathing of the veins results from either infiltration of their walls as from inflammatory processes or from cellular changes in the walls secondary to venous stasis. The extreme of this occurs with venous occlusion when the vein becomes a white, bloodless cord. Milder forms result in an opaque border to the blood column in a manner that has been called "halo ensheathing"[373] but it must be differentiated from fibrous cuffing that occurs in normal vessels as they

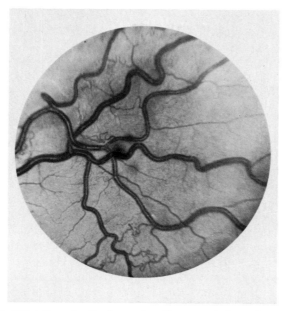

Figure 35 Dilatation of retinal vessels with congenital arteriovenous shunts. The fundi showed many small vessels connecting the arteries and veins.

emerge from the disc. An especially interesting incidence of retinal venous ensheathing occurs with multiple sclerosis,[557] suggesting a periphlebitis component to this enigmatic disease. The incidence of this ensheathing is estimated to be 10 to 26 per cent of all cases of multiple sclerosis.[277]

Arteriovenous (AV) Crossings

Retinal arteries generally cross superficial to the veins and the two are locally bound in a common adventitia. This sharing of the adventitia predisposes to venous occlusion with either sclerosis of the artery or congestion of the veins. It is, in fact, the common cause of tributary venous occlusion.

With sclerosis of the artery, the veins show at the AV crossing a more nearly right-angle branching, banking of blood, and occasionally dilatation of collaterals. To a certain degree these are normal senile changes but they become accentuated in conditions of decreased arterial flow, hyperviscosity of blood, and increased back pressure (glaucoma, papilledema, and orbital masses). Ominous signs pointing to threatened total occlusion are hemorrhages or fluoroangiographic evidence of leaks at the AV crossings. On the other hand, a slow development of venous obstruction may be compensated by dilatation of collateral vessels, bypassing the AV crossing or proliferating into the overlying vitreous (see p. 128). The former occurs asymptomatically and is a good sign but the latter entails a risk of vitreous hemorrhages which may be catastrophic.

Cotton-Wool Spots

Cotton-wool spots in the retina occur in a variety of vascular diseases including hypertension, embolic occlusion, anemia, and the collagenoses, and sometimes in senility, without apparent cause.[662] Although often interpreted erroneously as exudates, the spots actually represent swelling of the nerve fibers in consequence of microinfarcts.

The cotton-wool spots are easily identified by their white color, by their invariably superficial position in the retina (often covering the retinal vessels), and by their exclusive position in the posterior portions of the fundus (Fig. 36). They vary in size but are rarely bigger than one half the disc diameter and are usually much smaller. The size of the spot varies with the size of the obstructed arteriole; usually these obstructed vessels are of the order of 20 μ. The spots do not stain with fluorescein but small leaks and occasional hemorrhages are to be found in the vicinity along with an underlying area of avascularity.[585]

Sometimes mistaken for cotton-wool spots are patches of myelinated nerve fibers (Fig. 37). These, too, are white and have fimbriated edges

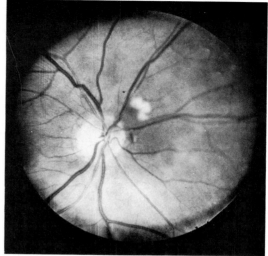

Figure 36 Solitary cotton-wool spot adjacent to disc.

The patient was a 60 year old man with hypertension but no ocular symptoms. Adjacent to the cotton-wool spot the retinal artery appeared constricted.

suggesting cotton but they may be easily distinguished by being larger (usually), overlapping the disc margins, obscuring the retinal vessels, and occurring in otherwise normal eyes.

Although cotton-wool spots are nonspecific in that they indicate merely arteriolar obstruction, they tend to predominate in some vasculopathies and not in others. They are especially conspicuous in lupus erythematosus[40, 456] and the collagenoses (dermatomyositis[162, 689] and scleroderma[386, 528]) in which hemorrhage and exudates may be minimal. Conversely, they tend to be relatively inconspicuous in diabetic retinopathy in which hemorrhages and exudate predominate.

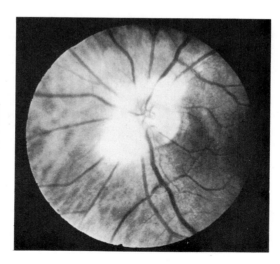

Figure 37 Myelination of nerve fibers. This is a normal variant that is sometimes mistaken for a cotton-wool spot or exudate.

With transient emboli, anemia, or carotid stenosis[324, 325] they may appear as solitary and sometimes large spots. With hypertension the number of cotton-wool spots parallels the hemorrhagic and exudative retinopathy.

Cotton-wool spots have been produced in animals by injection of latex and glass microspheres.[30, 35, 241] The experimental evidence corroborates the clinical impression of arteriolar obstruction in the 20 μ range. They appear within 24 to 48 hours after the obstruction and resolve in several weeks' time. In lupus erythematosus the coming and going of the spots has been plotted over a period of one year until the death of the patient.[67]

Cotton-wool spots may also occur on the disc but with vascular disease they are less conspicuous than with papilledema. In this latter case they are associated with a ring of hemorrhage and exudate in the peripapillary region, presenting the typical picture of florid papilledema (see p. 57).

Histologically, cotton-wool spots consist of focal swelling of the nerve fibers.[27] By photomicroscopy the swollen area typically contains spherical aggregates that resemble nuclei; hence, the lesions are called cytoid bodies (Fig. 38). They were, in fact, originally interpreted as swollen astrocytes[220] but Hortega silver stains[691] and electron microscopy[29, 35, 583] have shown them to be swollen nerve fibers with accumulations of mitochondria accounting for the nucleus-like

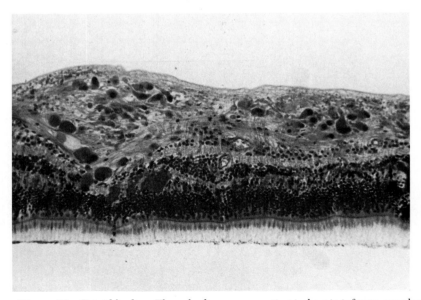

Figure 38 Cytoid bodies. These bodies, representing ischemic infarcts, are characterized by swelling and acellularity of the inner layers of the retina and the formation of round aggregates that have a superficial resemblance to cells. They are the histologic counterpart of the cotton-wool spots.

staining. Similar staining may occur with traumatic section of the nerve fibers and the swollen axones are then found to involve the proximal end of the neurites (that is, away from the disc), suggesting an abortive attempt at regeneration.[694] Similar changes occur in the spinal cord.[695]

Occasionally an obstructed vessel, or dilated collateral vessel, may be seen at the edge of the cytoid body. Its excessive basement membrane distinguishes it from a normal vessel.

Exudates

True exudates (in contrast to cotton-wool spots) present ophthalmoscopically as punctate yellowish white spots scattered throughout the fundus. Sometimes called hard, waxy, or fatty exudates they are most abundant at the posterior pole and often assume a radiating star figure about the macula (Fig. 39). They occur nonspecifically in any retinal vasculopathy that produces leaky vessels and are especially conspicuous in diabetes, hypertension, venous stasis, and vascular anomalies (von Hippel's angiomatosis, Coats' disease, and Leber's telangiectasis). On the other hand, exudate tends to be an inconspicuous feature in the retinopathy of the collagenoses unaccompanied by hypertension.

The exudate sometimes erupts posteriorly into the subretinal space spreading out to form yellowish, occasionally scintillating,

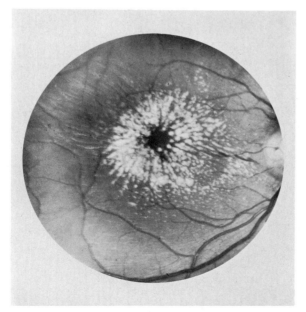

Figure 39 Star figure consisting of exudates about the macula.

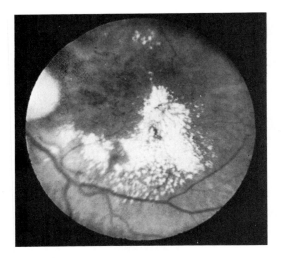

Figure 40 Conglomerate mass of exudate which has presumably erupted posteriorly into the subretinal space. The patient was a diabetic.

masses (Fig. 40). When these masses surround the central area they constitute what is known as circinate retinopathy.

Histologically this exudate consists initially of serum confined to the outer reticular layer of the retina (Fig. 41). The vertical orientation of Müller's fibers and of neurones restrains the lateral spread of the exudate, thus accounting for the characteristically punctate configuration of the spots seen ophthalmoscopically. Large aggregations of exudate occur only when the retina has been destroyed. The formation

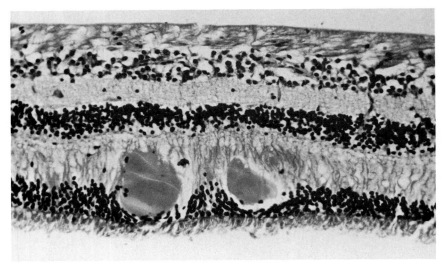

Figure 41 Two foci of exudate situated in the outer reticular layer of the retina. The patient was a diabetic.

of the star figure about the macula is due to the radiating fibers of Henle's layer which orient the spread of serum in a cartwheel manner.

The exclusive occurrence of exudate in the outer reticular layer and its absence from the inner layers is surprising. One possible explanation is its proximity to the deepest capillaries. Whatever the explanation, it seems to have a reciprocal relationship to the cotton-wool spots which occur in the same condition but which are found exclusively in the inner retinal layers.

The serous exudate either absorbs with minimal phagocytic activity or undergoes lipid metamorphosis with eventual phagocytosis. Clusters of lipid-containing cells may completely replace the exudates. The lipid metamorphosis and cellular reaction are conspicuous with serum that has erupted through the external limiting membrane into the subretinal area. This is especially common in diabetes and Coats' disease.

The exudative spots are easily confused ophthalmoscopically with the hyaline excrescences of Bruch's membrane called *drusen bodies* (Fig. 42). These are also yellowish dots that may be widely scattered throughout the fundus. Occasionally they form conglomerate masses in the central area to comprise one form of macular degeneration. Differentiation from exudate should present little difficulty because drusen are not associated with hemorrhage or other evidence of vasculopathy as occurs regularly with exudate. A further

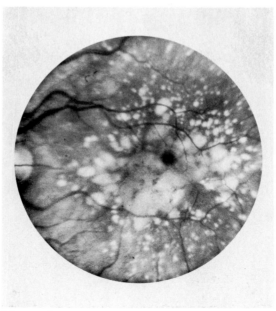

Figure 42 Massive drusen which are often mistaken for exudates but are actually hyaline excrescences of Bruch's membrane.

point in differentiation is the pigment clumping that frequently surrounds drusen. Fluoroangiography provides a means for definitive differentiation. Drusen fluoresce early and intensely whereas exudates not only fail to light up but actually obscure the background fluorescence.

Hemorrhages

Hemorrhages in the fundus may present as intraretinal or extraretinal extravasations and, like exudates, owe their appearances to the physical restraints of the surrounding tissue.

Intraretinal hemorrhages may be flame-shaped, punctate, or focally massive, depending on their depth within the retina. Flame-shaped or splinter hemorrhages are superficial and owe their configuration to the horizontally coursing nerve fibers (Fig. 43). Punctate ("dot and blot") hemorrhages are deeper in the retina and owe their configuration to the lateral restraints imposed by the vertically coursing nerve fibers. The massive hemorrhages are most superficially situated between the internal limiting membrane and the nerve fiber layer.

The type of intraretinal hemorrhage has some, though limited, pathogenetic significance. The flame-shaped hemorrhages are most

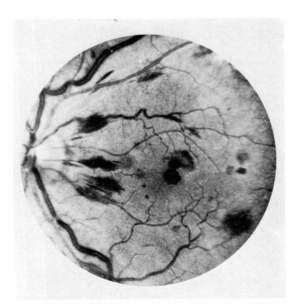

Figure 43 Predominantly flame-shaped hemorrhages.

The patient was a 58 year old woman with macroglobulinemia and a blood viscosity of 25.

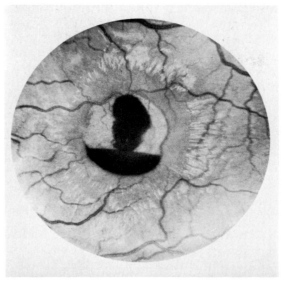

Figure 44 Focally massive hemorrhage overlying the macula. Noteworthy is the tendency of the red cells to settle and thereby to form a fluid level overlain by serum. (The fine lines radiating from the macula are light reflexes from the surface of the retina.)

The patient was a 26 year old man with aplastic anemia and thrombocytopenia.

suggestive of diffuse vascular disease and predominate in hypertension although they can occur in many conditions including hyperviscosity syndromes. With papilledema they form a characteristic corona about the disc. The punctate hemorrhages point especially to capillary disease and predominate in diabetic retinopathy. Focally massive hemorrhages occur with any of several diseases but are especially common with subarachnoid hemorrhage, leukemia, and diabetes.

The peculiar nature of these focally massive hemorrhages warrants special comment. They are erroneously called subhyaloid or pre-retinal hemorrhages. Probably arising from the radial peripapillary capillaries and dissecting up the internal limiting membrane they find little resistance to lateral spread. In consequence, they form large circular masses of blood in the region overlying the macula or between the macula and the disc (Fig. 44). The blood in these masses remains curiously unclotted so that as the patient sits up, the red cells sink to the lower half and present a fluid level with yellowish serum above.

Venous obstruction produces a fundus picture characterized by extensive flame-shaped hemorrhages involving the entire fundus (see venous obstruction, p. 127). Except when they are covered by the hemorrhages, the dilated veins can be seen emerging from the hemorrhagic background. The common site for obstruction of the central retinal vein is at the lamina cribrosa in the nerve head but tributary occlusions occur at arteriovenous junctions. With tributary occlusion, the hemorrhages have a fan-shaped distribution in the retina radiating out from the point of an AV crossing. They are not as massive nor accompanied by as much congestion as is the case with central vein occlusion.

It may be stated categorically that extensive hemorrhages within the retina are always of venous origin whereas hemorrhages in the vitreous may be of venous origin or, more usually, of neovasculogenic origin. In either case they are not of arterial origin and thereby differ from cerebral hemorrhages, which are believed to result from arterial blow-outs or encephalomalacia.[291]

Hemorrhages occurring with tributary arterial occlusion are infrequent. They are then small and situated on the border of the infarcted area.

Hemorrhages with a white center are called Roth spots and are classically associated with subacute bacterial endocarditis (Fig. 45). There is little question that they do occur with this disease,[150, 372] but they are not as diagnostic as was at one time believed.[595] They may, in fact, be found with retinal hemorrhages of any etiology and have been especially observed in leukemia.[7, 129]

Hemorrhages anterior to the retina arise chiefly from the neovascular proliferations which have extended into the vitreous cavity

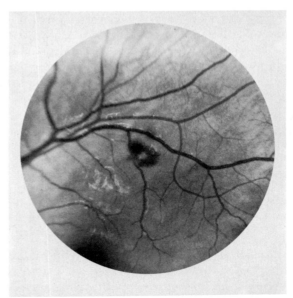

Figure 45 Roth spot (hemorrhage with white center) in a patient with subacute bacterial endocarditis.

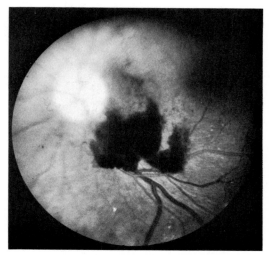

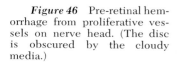 **Figure 46** Pre-retinal hem-
orrhage from proliferative ves-
sels on nerve head. (The disc
is obscured by the cloudy
media.)

*The patient was a 39 year
old woman who had had diabetes for 39 years.*

either from the nerve head (Fig. 46) where the internal limiting membrane is least well developed or from the retina where the internal limiting membrane has been perforated. The walls of these neovascular channels are extremely thin and leaky. The blood may diffuse throughout the vitreous or be confined to local streaks, depending on the turgor of the vitreous body. The conditions causing these pre-retinal hemorrhages are primarily those which predispose to neovascular proliferations ("retinitis proliferans") through the internal limiting membrane. Diabetes is by far the most common (see p. 56).

One cause of vitreous hemorrhage not dependent on prior neovasculogenesis is subarachnoid hemorrhage. Here streamers of blood can often be seen extending from the nerve head into the vitreous, suggesting a direct extravasation from the subarachnoid space about the optic nerve (Fig. 47).[100, 447] Histologic studies have not, however, shown any such continuity of blood through the nerve, and how it gets into the eye is a question.[481]

A further cause of vitreous hemorrhage not dependent on retinal vascular disease is that which occurs with ruptures of the retina. These ruptures may occur spontaneously, especially in myopic eyes, and sometimes precede a detachment of the retina. For this reason ophthalmologists insist on following patients with spontaneous vitreous hemorrhages carefully and rely on indirect ophthalmoscopy in searching the retinal periphery for holes in the retina.

Subretinal hemorrhages may arise from the retinal vessels by direct extension through the external limiting membrane but this is less common than hemorrhage from the choriocapillaris. Subretinal hemorrhages are dark red to black in color, generally large, and cause measurable elevation of the retina (Fig. 48). The feature of subretinal hemorrhages which distinguishes them from other types is the liability to phagocytosis and lipid metamorphosis. Thus they soon form

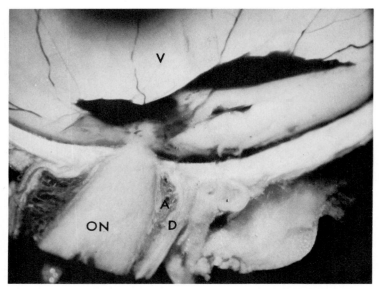

Figure 47 Gross specimen of the transected eye from a patient with subarachnoid hemorrhage. *ON*, optic nerve; *A*, arachnoid; *D*, dura; *V*, vitreous space. Blood can be seen in the subarachnoid space about the optic nerve and within the eye but not between the two.

yellowish white masses that either suggest tumor or form circular masses called circinate retinopathy. Such hemorrhages and post-hemorrhagic conditions are especially frequent with diabetes and Coats' disease.

The subretinal hemorrhages arising from the retina are not to be confused with those that give rise to disciform degeneration of the macula. These latter arise from neovascular buds of the choriocapillaris and are the indirect result of ruptures of Bruch's membrane. The hemorrhages usually occur without apparent provocation but an especially severe case has been reported in association with anticoagulation.[194] Recurrent bleeding from these neovascular proliferations and the subsequent organization produce masses that destroy the overlying retina.[235] Termed *disciform degeneration of the macula,* it is one of the more common causes of blindness in older persons. It occurs with angioid streaks (see p. 96) but is not otherwise known to be associated with systemic disease.

The symptoms caused by retinal hemorrhage depend entirely on the coexistent involvement of the macula or of the visual axis. Small hemorrhages overlying the fovea will result in disproportionately severe loss of vision whereas extensive hemorrhagic retinopathy which spares the fovea, as occurs in hypertensive retinopathy for instance, may be entirely asymptomatic. In the vitreous, massive hemorrhages will reduce vision to light perception but small hemorrhages will simply cause showers of floating opacities.

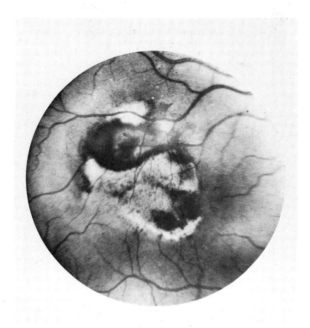

Figure 48 Subretinal hemorrhage undergoing metaplasia.

The patient was a 61 year old woman who developed sudden loss of vision in the eye. The appearance is typical of the entity known as disciform degeneration of the macula which follows hemorrhage from the choriocapillaris.

Hemorrhages in the retina absorb more slowly than in most tissues where phagocytosis is active. Occasionally small hemorrhages leave a small gliotic scar or irregularity of the light reflex that can be seen ophthalmologically, but usually the hemorrhages disappear entirely in the course of a few weeks without leaving any significant residue. When the hemorrhage is massive, however, as after a central vein obstruction, the retina may develop a correspondingly massive gliosis and eventual detachment. A further complication, after central vein occlusion, is the development of a particularly malignant "hemorrhagic glaucoma."

Vascular Proliferative Retinopathy (Retinitis Proliferans)

Under conditions that are only partially understood, blood vessels grow from the retina into the vitreous space where they form either rich plexuses lying on the surface of the retina or arborizing fans extending into the center of the vitreous space. While undergoing regression in one area and being replaced by acellular connective tissue they tend to proliferate in another area to run an inexorable course of cicatrization of the vitreous and often blindness.

The customary name retinitis proliferans is especially inappropriate since the condition is neither an inflammation nor a proliferation of the retina. Actually vessels do not proliferate within the retina (except under conditions of severe necrosis) but rather into the vitreous. The common ophthalmoscopic impression of retinal neovasculogenesis is either a misinterpretation of dilated preformed vessels (shunt vessels) within the retina or vessels in the vitreous lying on the surface of the retina.

The newly formed vessels in the vitreous have extremely thin walls and consequently leak serum (as seen dramatically by fluoroangiography) and blood. The hemorrhages occur precipitously and are often massive. They in turn lead to further neovascularization so that a vicious cycle is set up whereby the vascular proliferation leads to hemorrhage and the hemorrhage leads to further proliferation. Fortunately many cases remit with partial resolution of the proliferative tissue.

The systemic conditions responsible for vascular proliferative retinopathy include primarily diabetes (see p. 83). The vessels derive chiefly from the nerve head and form an epipapillary plexus that may give rise to recurrent hemorrhages. It is practically always bilateral and comprises the most dreaded type of diabetic retinopathy. Sickle cell disease, especially SC variety, induces a vascular proliferation that differs from that of diabetes in coming from the periphery of the retina rather than from the disc area. Other obliterative processes, such as Eales' disease (see p. 116), may induce similar vascular fans arising from the periphery. Venous compression at an arteriovenous junction is sometimes associated with bypass extension of vessels into the vitreous. (See also Retrolental Fibroplasia, p. 117.)

To understand the pathogenesis of vascular proliferative retinopathy one should recall that the vitreous is in fact a connective tissue space with a uniquely rich amount of ground substance and a relative paucity of collagen. It is separated from the retina by a basement membrane called the internal limiting membrane. This latter, as its normal function, appears to prevent the extension of blood vessels into the vitreous. However, it is extremely tenuous overlying the disc and is prone to rupture at the sites of contact with the major blood vessels of the retina. These are the two sites from which neovasculogenesis occurs in proliferative retinopathy. Once the internal limiting membrane is perforated the blood vessels grow freely in the connective tissue space of the vitreous. The pathogenesis of vascular proliferative retinopathy revolves, therefore, about those conditions which make the internal limiting membrane invadable. In diabetes the basis is obscure[43] but in most of the other conditions it seems to be local obliterative vascular disease.

Papilledema

While meaning literally swelling of the optic nerve head, papilledema has come to apply specifically to that type of swelling associated with stasis rather than with inflammation. Thus by common usage papilledema refers to swelling from increased intracranial pressure, often called "choked disc," or from the venous back pressure (orbital masses and vascular obstruction). The swelling with inflammation, on the other hand, is customarily included in the term *papillitis*. The two conditions are usually distinguished by the effect on vision. Papilledema, per se, causes no reduction in vision except in severe instances in which the edema extends to the macula. Papillitis, by contrast, reduces vision markedly even when the edema of the disc is minimal.

Chronic papilledema is characterized simply by obscuration of the disc margins, elevation of the nerve head, and, at times, venous congestion. Acute papilledema causes, in addition, multiple flame-shaped hemorrhages and cotton-wool spots on and about the disc (Figs. 49, 50, and 51).

Edema of the nerve head occurs with ischemic optic neuropathy and to some extent with occlusive venous disease and with hypertensive retinopathy. However, the chief cause of papilledema is elevation of intracranial pressure or orbital masses. Since the meningeal spaces about the optic nerve are continuous with those about the brain, they reflect the intracranial pressure directly. Papilledema is also an occasional manifestation of pulmonary emphysema[38, 218, 600] and cystic fibrosis.[38] The hypercapnia may exert its effect through local dilatation of the papillary capillaries[618] rather than through increased intracranial pressure.

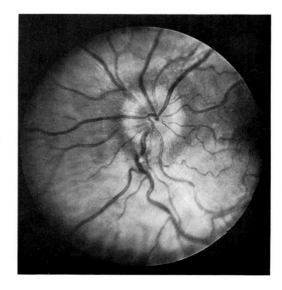

Figure 49 Mild papilledema.

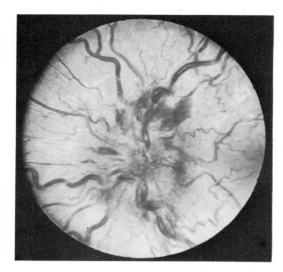

Figure 50   Moderate papilledema.

   The ophthalmoscopic appearance of the papilledema and associated symptoms may give some clue as to the etiology. Papilledema
resulting from increased intracranial pressure presents a cylindric
protrusion with preservation of the physiologic cup and often concen-
tric ripples in the adjacent retina. The hemorrhages and cotton-wool
spots, when present, are limited to the disc and to the immediately
peripapillary region. Headaches are the rule but vision may be remarkably unaffected. By contrast, the papilledema with hypertension is
accompanied by a diffuse edema extending into the retina and associated with widespread hemorrhages and exudate. Similarly, the

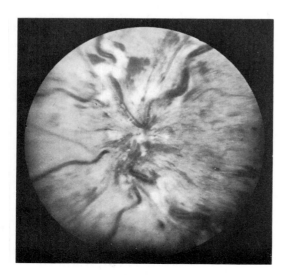

Figure 51   Severe papilledema.

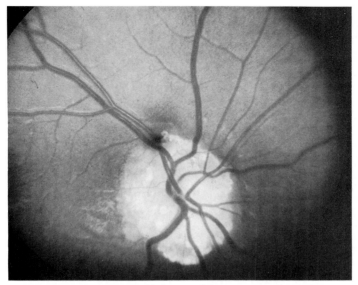

Figure 52   Drusen (pseudopapilledema) of the nerve head. Characteristic are the white, translucent bodies embedded in the nerve head.

papilledema with venous occlusive disease is associated with widespread but often massive hemorrhages. Both conditions are associated with a degree of visual loss depending on the involvement of the macula.

Differentiation of true papilledema from the pseudopapilledema of hyperopia or from deep-lying hyaline bodies within the papilla (drusen) is a real problem in borderline cases (Fig. 52).* The presence of spontaneous venous pulsation on the disc, as occurs frequently in normal eyes, rules out papilledema. Leakage of fluorescein from the disc region points to true papilledema (Fig. 53),[280] but unfortunately fluoroangiography fails to help in just those cases which are borderline. Enlargement of the blind spot on field testing is highly subjective and unreliable. Perhaps the best criterion for differentiation, at least for the sophisticated observer, is the ophthalmoscopic detection of abnormally dilated capillaries on the disc. With true papilledema these look like microaneurysms.

Ischemic optic neuropathy is characterized by swelling of the disc, considerable loss of vision, and often sectorial pallor of the nerve head (see p. 107). The pallor, when present, the absence of pain, and the age of the patient suggest the differentiation from papillitis and

*The term *drusen* applies, unfortunately, to two distinct entities. Drusen of the nerve head are not to be confused with the excrescences of Bruch's membrane which are also called drusen.

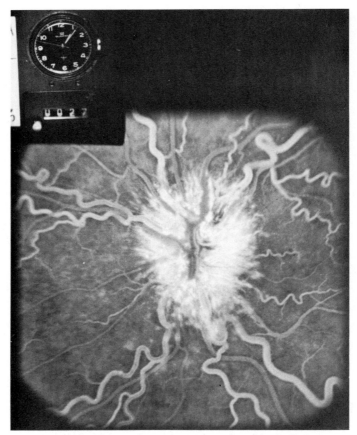

Figure 53 Fluoroangiogram from a patient with mild papilledema. Noteworthy are the conspicuous dilatation of the small vessels, the tortuosity of the large vessels, and the leakage of dye from the nerve head.

papilledema. However, this differentiation is not always clear-cut, and fluoroangiography does not afford much help.

Longitudinal sections of optic nerves with papilledema show swelling of the nerve head with a surprisingly sharp and characteristically S-shaped border with the retina (Fig. 54). The nerve may project one or more millimeters into the vitreous space and displace the retina laterally, forming wrinkles of the posterior retinal surface.

Diffuse Opacity and Cherry Red Spot

Diffuse opacification of the retina generally points to cloudy swelling of the ganglion cells and is most dense posteriorly, corresponding to the population of these cells. Since the ganglion cells are absent in the center of the fovea, a central "hole" escapes this opacity and transmits the red choroidal reflex as a cherry red spot that contrasts with the white background.

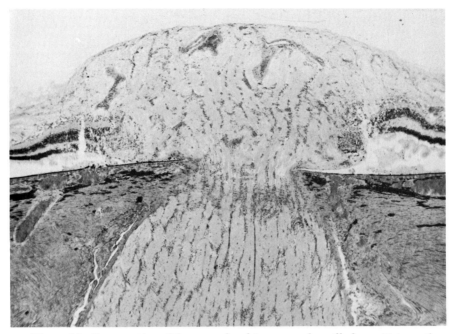

Figure 54 Cross-section of the nerve head in a case of papilledema. Noteworthy are the swelling of the nerve substance, the dilatation of vessels, and the lateral displacement of the adjacent retina. (To be compared with the normal nerve head illustrated in Figure 31.)

The two conditions which are classically associated with diffuse opacification of the retina are retinal artery occlusion and certain storage diseases.

The opacity with central artery occlusion is due to cloudy swelling of the ganglion cells and to associated edema. It disappears as the ganglion cells die and does not occur at all if the ganglion cells have been destroyed prior to the occlusion.

The opacity of the sphingolipidoses is due to accumulation of the material, usually lipid, in the ganglion cells (Fig. 55). It is most familiar in Tay-Sachs disease, in which it is a constant feature, but it also occurs in other gangliosidoses and to a less obvious degree in other lipid-storage diseases (metachromatic leukodystrophy,[110] Niemann-Pick's disease,[464] Gaucher's disease, and Farber's lipogranulomatosis[112]) and rarely in the mucopolysaccharidoses.[257]

Opacification of the retina with a cherry red spot may occur rarely in otherwise normal eyes and is then asymptomatic.

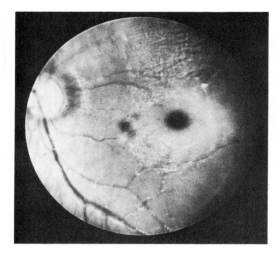

Figure 55 Opacification of the central retina and a cherry red spot in Tay-Sachs disease. (The dark spot on the nasal edge of the opacity is a photographic artifact, and the fine linear streaks above the opacity are light reflexes from the surface of the retina.)

Optic Atrophy

Pallor of the disc is used synonymously with optic atrophy to indicate an inferred loss of nerve fibers (Fig. 56). Actually the disc becomes pale through loss of its capillaries and is therefore only an indirect consequence of optic atrophy. It is a relative index showing considerable variation among individuals and becoming manifest only after a delay of weeks or months depending on whether the site of the lesion is close to or away from the globe.

Optic atrophy is rather unsatisfactorily divided into primary and secondary depending on the amount of glial or other tissue on the nerve head in addition to the pallor. Lesions of either the retinal gan-

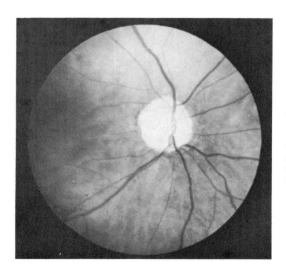

Figure 56 Pallor of the disc indicating optic atrophy.

The patient was a 76 year old man who had become completely blind six months previously after a massive gastrointestinal hemorrhage.

glion cells or the retrobulbar portion of the optic nerve produce simply a white disc with the normal sharp edges. Lesions of the nerve head itself, such as occur following papilledema or papillitis, are associated with an overlay of glial tissue producing a grayish white color and some fuzziness of the disc margins. Gliomas of the optic nerve are especially apt to produce a prominent gliosis with optic atrophy while hyaline excrescences (drusen) within the nerve produce characteristically translucent bodies in association with the optic atrophy.

The causes of optic atrophy are legion and most are beyond the scope of this text. Vascular lesions may produce either primary or secondary optic atrophy, depending on whether they are situated away from or on the disc. Ischemic optic neuropathy and retinal artery occlusion are the common vascular accidents. Next in importance, perhaps, are the demyelinative disorders which may also produce either a primary or secondary optic atrophy, but in cases of primary optic atrophy intracranial tumors are always suspect until proved otherwise, since the region of the chiasm and adjacent optic nerves is a relatively silent area neurologically. Moreover, tumors of the sellar and parasellar region are common.

The histopathology of optic atrophy consists of loss of the myelinated fibers in the optic nerve, with consequent collapse of the fibrovascular scaffolding, loss of the nerve fibers from the inner layer of the retina, and disappearance of the ganglion cells of the retina. Since the optic nerve fibers are the axones of the ganglion cells, both disappear with optic atrophy, and it is often not possible to ascertain from the pathology alone whether the primary lesion is in the retina or in the nerve

Chorioretinal Lesions

Most, if not all, choroidal vasculopathies of clinical significance involve the overlying pigment epithelium and retina. They are best considered collectively, therefore, as chorioretinal lesions. What one sees clinically are chiefly the secondary phenomena while the primary vasculopathy is obscured by the overlying tissue changes.

Diffuse attenuation of the pigment epithelium occurs regularly with age and may, in darkly complected individuals, lead to the familiar tessellated fundus characterized by a mosaic of choroidal vessels and interstitial pigment (Fig. 57). This is sometimes interpreted as diffuse choroidal sclerosis but such a conclusion lacks histologic confirmation.

With attenuation of the pigment or with absence of the pigment epithelium, the choroidal vessels stand out unusually well by fluoroangiography.[314]

Circumscribed loss of the pigment epithelium with consequent focal exposure of the choroid occurs in various patterns but is seen

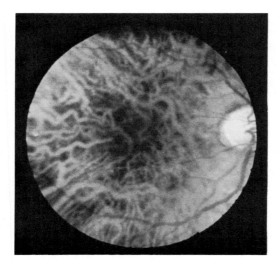

Figure 57 Senile tessellation. Noteworthy is the unusual visibility of the choroidal vessels.

The patient was a 73 year old woman whose choroidal vessels had become visible through attenuation of the pigment epithelium.

most commonly in a circular zone encompassing the macula. It is then known as areolar macular degeneration (erroneously referred to as central areolar sclerosis) and is a frequent cause of impaired vision affecting both eyes. It is often hereditary. The pathogenesis of this and other types of loss of the pigment epithelium is obscure but a popular conviction is that it depends on obliteration of the underlying choriocapillaris. Absence of the choriocapillaris has, in fact, been confirmed fluoroangiographically and by injection of an enucleated eye with the degeneration,[24, 615] but the question remains whether the choriocapillary occlusion was the cause or the result of the areolar degeneration.

Chorioretinal degenerations usually involve much more than simple loss of the pigment epithelium. The commonest lesions (whether they be post-inflammatory, vascular, or primarily degenerative), present irregular clumps of black pigment, white scar tissue, exposed sclera, and loss of retinochoroidal landmarks (Fig. 58). A few remaining choroidal vessels may be recognized in the base of the lesion.

The common inflammatory disease causing chorioretinal scars is toxoplasmosis but other alleged or proved causes include cytomegalic inclusion disease, congenital syphilis, and histoplasmosis. Vascular occlusion in the choroid produces pigmented areas (Elschnig spots)[74, 388, 482] and possibly accounts for the common degenerative foci in the mid-periphery that are termed pavement (cobble-stone) degeneration. In sickle cell disease these foci have been called the black sunset sign.[677] Clumping of pigment over a sclerosed choroidal vessel often forms a linear streak known as the Siegrist sign.[593]

The choroidal arteries participate in many of the systemic arteritides. Involvement with polyarteritis has been frequently reported

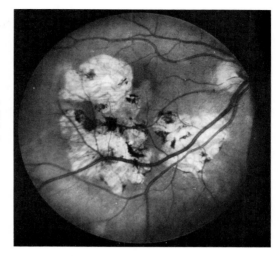

Figure 58 Foci of chorio-retinal degeneration presenting clumps of pigment and a white background of scar tissue, choroidal vessels, and sclera.

pathologically[61, 223, 258, 259, 313] but rarely clinically.[62, 689] The arteries have also shown the typical pathology of thrombotic thrombocytopenia[467] but, surprisingly, have rarely been involved with temporal arteritis despite the involvement of the parent ciliary vessels.[482]

Detachment of Retina and of Pigment Epithelium

The common idiopathic detachment of the retina is a local process resulting from a hole in the retina and consequent separation of the photoreceptors from the pigment epithelium. Secondary detachment of the retina may occur, however, when serum exudes from the choriocapillaris, penetrating the pigment epithelium and peeling off the retina. A mild degree of this occurs in hypertension, diabetes, and various vasculopathies but it is most severe in eclampsia, thrombotic thrombocytopenia, and nephritis. These cause characteristically bilateral and reversible detachment of the retina in the lower half of the fundus.[248, 388, 482, 503] Yet it may be asymptomatic since loss of the upper field, corresponding to detachment of the lower retina, causes little functional impairment.

The pathogenesis of these detachments of the pigment epithelium and retina appears to be obstruction of the choriocapillaris or of the small vessels connected with the choriocapillaris. This is a constant finding with serous detachments accompanying systemic vascular disease and may be produced experimentally by injecting microspheres into the choroid by way of the vortex veins.[116]

Focal detachments of the retina and pigment epithelium occur with several entities that carry descriptive names and may be of vascular origin but in which the pathogenesis is actually obscure.

Most common is central serous retinopathy that consists of serous exudate from one or several points of the choriocapillaris. The serum elevates the pigment epithelium and erupts into the subretinal space. This occurs predominately in young adult males, affects one or both eyes, and is frequently recurrent. Since the central area is affected preferentially, vision is considerably impaired, but as long as the serum remains confined beneath the pigment epithelium, the photoreceptors remain intact and vision returns to normal within a few weeks.

The ophthalmoscopic changes of central serous retinopathy are often subtle and present no more than a relatively flat elevation of the retina and loss of the foveolar light reflex. Fluoroangiography, however, reveals a sharply circumscribed zone of detachment when the serum is beneath the pigment epithelium and, more significantly, one or more points of choriocapillary leak. When the serum erupts through the pigment epithelium, the fluorescence presents a more diffuse stain.

SUMMARY

Narrowing and irregularity of the retinal arteries occur with hypertension but evaluation must take into account the anatomic and optical variations as well as the diffuse narrowing which occurs with tissue atrophy and some of the retinal abiotrophies. Tortuosity of the arteries is primarily a senile occurrence but is also seen congenitally and in association with coarctation of the aorta and congenital heart disease.

Congestion and tortuosity of the veins occur with venous obstructive disease and are often suggestive of hyperviscosity syndromes. Tributary venous obstruction is most evident at arteriovenous crossings where the artery and vein are bound in a common adventitia. Increasing rigidity of the arterial wall may precipitate the venous obstruction.

Cotton-wool spots are microinfarcts of the retina which appear histologically as cytoid bodies. They are situated in the nerve fiber (inner) layer of the retina. Although occurring with any obstructive vascular disease, they predominate in the non-hypertensive collagenoses. Exudates, on the other hand, appear as yellowish dots and consist of serum in the outer reticular (deep) layer of the retina. They owe their configuration to the physical constraints of the adjacent retina. Exudates occur in all vascular retinopathies but are especially conspicuous in hypertension and diabetes.

Hemorrhages have different configurations and to some extent differing etiologic significance, depending on their site in the retina. Flame-shaped hemorrhages predominate in hypertension whereas punctate hemorrhages predominate in diabetes, but there is considerable overlap between these two diseases and other vasculopathies. Massive hemorrhages in the retina suggest venous occlusive disease while massive hemorrhages into the vitreous suggest either prior neovasculogenesis from the retina or subarachnoid hemorrhage. Subretinal hemorrhages result from either extension of retinal hemorrhage or neovasculogenesis from the choroid.

Proliferative vascular retinopathy is an ingrowth of vessels into the vitreous and is especially characteristic of diabetes. Although progressing and remitting, often at the same time, it frequently leads to massive intraocular hemorrhage with catastrophic scar formation and a type of retinal detachment that is refractory to treatment.

Edema of the disc results from increased intracranial pressure (papilledema) or inflammation (papillitis) or from occlusive vascular disease (ischemic optic neuropathy) of the papilla. The effect on vision and the association with pain are helpful but not altogether reliable criteria for the differentiation.

Diffuse opacity of the retina such as occurs with arterial occlusion results from cloudy swelling of the ganglion cells in the retina while that which occurs with the sphingolipidoses is due to lipid storage in the ganglion cells. The cherry red spot is the contrast visualization of the red choroid through that portion of the retina which has no ganglion cells.

Optic atrophy results from loss of nerve fibers, whether the lesions be in the ganglion cells of the retina or in the optic nerve itself. The characteristic pallor of the disc is due to the secondary attrition of the capillaries and follows the optic atrophy by a time interval that varies according to the distance of the lesion from the papilla.

Chorioretinal lesions, whether they be of vasculogenic, degenerative, or inflammatory origin, are characterized by pigmentary and cicatricial changes in which direct visualization of the vascular lesions is rarely possible. Detachment of the retina and pigment epithelium follows exudation from the choriocapillaris and occurs with several local and systemic vasculopathies. It is not to be confused, however, with the common detachment of the retina which results from a tear in the retina and is not associated with systemic disease.

CHAPTER 4

SUBJECTIVE SYMPTOMS AND VISUAL FIELD ABNORMALITIES

Blackouts

Blackouts (amaurosis fugax) are cardinal signs of retinal or optic nerve ischemia, or more precisely of hypoxia.[11, 83] They occur with low blood pressure, are sometimes orthostatically induced, and may be bilateral or unilateral. Unilateral blackouts are especially suggestive of carotid stenosis[57, 206] or of the aortic arch syndrome. The blackout is described variously as a "blur," "shade," or general dimming of vision and is apt to begin in the lower field. Rarely does it last more than 10 minutes, and recovery follows the reverse order of its onset. With ischemic optic neuropathy (see p. 107), several attacks of amaurosis may precede a permanent blindness. On the other hand, attacks may recur for months or years without permanent residua. Neither the frequency nor the duration of the attacks gives any indication of the ultimate prognosis.[453]

The combination of blackouts in one eye and hemiplegia on the opposite side of the body is a classic sign of carotid stenosis,[206] subject to confirmation by arteriography. Initially these symptoms were interpreted as simple ischemic episodes due to impaired circulation but the observation of moving emboli during the blackouts indicates that some and probably many cases are of embolic origin.[204, 328, 453] Yet blackouts are not always obviously ischemic in origin. They may occur with intracranial tumors and with papilledema and may be seen especially in young women without apparent cause.[96, 206, 453]

Amaurosis fugax was at one time attributed to spasm of the retinal arteries and was sometimes attributed to migraine.[86] The diminutive muscular coat of these arteries and the lack of other evidence for migraine makes this explanation unlikely.[453]

68

Photopsia and Scintillating Scotomas

Photopsias are the subjective flashes of light often called "seeing stars" in the popular jargon. They may arise from peripheral retinal stimulation and are then most commonly due to traction on the retina from vitreous pull with movements of the eye or from tears of the internal limiting membrane. At times they indicate hemorrhages in the retina. In the presence of an old detachment of the retina, the photopsias may be persistent and annoying even when the eye is blind. Photopsia arising in the central nervous system occurs most typically with occipital stimulation, especially from vascular lesions, and is then often projected into a hemianopic field. A relatively organized form of photopsia is the picket-fence scintillation characteristic of migraine (p. 150)[16] but seen occasionally with arteriovenous anomalies in the occipital area.

The scintillating scotomas of vascular lesions are characteristically projected to the field contralateral to the cerebral lesion. They are typically in constant motion or off and on, sometimes colored, and often likened to fireworks or lightning flashes. Less commonly the subjective phenomena are formed images, occasionally reenacting familiar scenes and events. They may be pleasant or frightening but, in general, the more complex and the less stereotyped they are the less they localize the site of the lesion. Indeed, the complex hallucinations seem to be less of an ictal manifestation than the release of an inherent activity once the normal inhibitory influences are removed.[102]

Metamorphopsia

Metamorphopsia is a distortion of the image in the central portion of the visual field. It is often described as a blur but specific inquiry reveals that the blur consists of a jog in straight lines or distortion of letters. Metamorphopsia is always a sign of macular disease and is especially characteristic of macular degeneration.

Floating Opacities

Floating opacities or muscae volitantes are the black spots that move with eye movements. They are due to specks in the vitreous and are to a certain extent normal residua of the embryonic vitreous. When marked, and especially when showers of them appear suddenly, they suggest hemorrhage into the vitreous with or without rupture of the retina. They are sometimes a forerunner of retinal detachment.

Scotomas

A scotoma is a discrete blind area in the visual field and differs from a constricted field defect which extends from the periphery.

Central scotomas impair visual acuity and, while occurring with various lesions, are most suggestive of macular disease or retrobulbar neuritis. Eccentric scotomas do not impair vision and may be unnoticed by the patient. Homonymous and symmetric paracentral scotomas in the two eyes point to a posterior occipital lesion and are usually indicative of small infarcts (p. 149).

Visual acuity is an index of the visual functions in the central portion of the visual field. It is customarily measured by reading letters on a Snellen chart in which the normal 20/20 vision indicates an ability to read at 20 feet (the numerator) what a normal person can read at 20 feet (the denominator). The acuity of 20/200, on the other hand, means that at 20 feet the observer can read only what a normal person does at 200 feet. Further reduction in vision is usually recorded in progressive terms as: counting fingers at so and so many feet; light projection; light perception; and nil vision.

Hemianopia

Hemianopia means literally half-sightedness and is typified by the visual field loss on one entire side of the vertical meridian. Actually the term is used for hemianopsias that are less than complete and *quadranopia* is the term for field defects that may be only approximately quadrantal. Homonymous hemianopia is the condition in which the visual field defect is on the same (that is, right or left) side in both eyes (Fig. 59). This invariably indicates a lesion of the visual pathways somewhere between the chiasm and the occipital pole. Further topologic localization is determined by the associated symptoms (p. 150). Bitemporal hemianopia, on the other hand, refers to a blindness in both temporal visual fields and points to a chiasmal lesion that has interrupted the crossing fibers (Fig. 60). It is most characteristic of pituitary or hypothalamic lesions. Less common and less

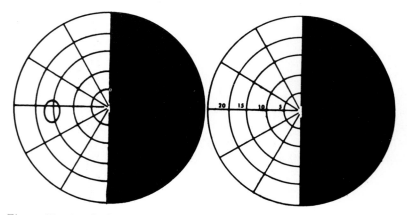

Figure 59 A right homonymous hemianopia indicates a left-sided lesion somewhere between the chiasm and posterior pole of the occiput.

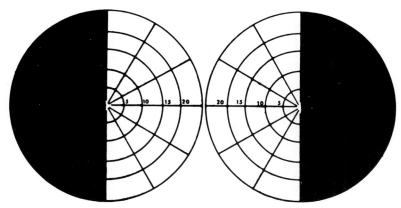

Figure 60   A bitemporal hemianopia indicates a lesion of the chiasm.

easily explained are the binasal hemianopias that have been reported with tumors, optochiasmatic arachnoiditis, and hydrocephalus.[228] The assumption is that they result from pressure of the carotid or anterior cerebral arteries against the lateral walls of the chiasm or optic nerves.[345] Some cases may merely represent the atrophy of papilledema.[342] In any event they do not result in the clean-cut hemianopias such as one sees in the bitemporal counterpart.

A common error is to assume that the dividing line of hemianopia passes through the nerve head. In fact, it passes through the fovea. There is no anatomic landmark for this in the retina but the reference points are sharply separated functionally at the chiasmal decussation and in the cerebrum.

Another frequent misconception is that hemianopia reduces the visual acuity. The recordable acuity is normal with one half the visual field. Reduction in the measured acuity means either that more than a hemianopia is present or that there is some additional cause for the loss of acuity.

Altitudinal hemianopia warrants special mention because of its frequent association with vascular lesions. The visual field defect of altitudinal hemianopia is demarcated by a horizontal line that corresponds to the horizontal raphé in the retina (Fig. 61). Its anatomic basis is either the retinal vasculature which has a sharp demarcation between upper and lower vessels or a functional separation at the optic foramen where the upper and lower nerve fibers are separated by the macular fibers. Altitudinal hemianopia occurs especially with vascular lesions in the retina (branch occlusions of the retinal artery) or with ischemic optic neuropathy. It also is seen with glaucoma and other lesions of the nerve head or optic foramen.

The symptoms produced by hemianopia may be surprisingly slight unless the central area is involved. The patient then complains typically of difficulty in reading. With right-sided hemianopia, he must read haltingly since he cannot scan successive words, whereas

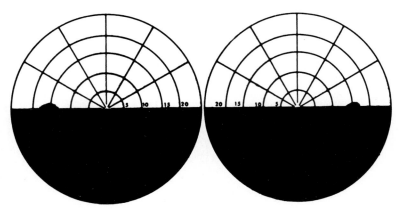

Figure 61 Altitudinal hemianopia usually indicates a lesion in the retina or optic nerve. It is rarely as complete as here indicated.

with left hemianopia he can read any one line with normal rapidity but loses his place on trying to find successive lines. Patients with hemianopia that spares the central area feel little incapacitation, even when they admit to bumping into objects on the affected side, and are apt to be dangerously overconfident in their ability to drive a car.

Bilateral homonymous hemianopia causes complete blindness; that resulting from lesions in the occiput differs from that of lesions in the optic nerves, chiasm, and tracts in the absence of optic atrophy and the retention of normal pupillary reactions.

Cortical blindness in man differs from that of monkeys and of all lower animals in that *all* vision is lost. The phylogeny of the visual systems has witnessed a progressive transfer of visual functions from the tectum of the brain stem to the cerebrum. In reptiles and birds, vision is entirely a mesencephalic function. Only in the human species has it been totally transferred to the cerebrum.

Cluster Headaches

Of obscure but probably vascular origin are the severe, unilateral headaches that are variously called cluster headaches, Horton's histaminic cephalalgia,[336, 337] and migrainous neuralgia.[291] They occur in unpredictable periods, affect predominantly middle-aged persons, are characterized by pain in and about the eye, congestion of the conjunctiva, and rhinorrhea, and are accompanied in from 5 to 20 per cent of the patients by transient or permanent Horner's syndrome.[411, 535, 548] The attacks frequently occur at night, wakening the patient one to two hours after he has fallen asleep and lasting from one half to several hours. The onset and termination are frequently abrupt. The headaches are apt to occur in clusters and then cease for several months without apparent reason.

The pathogenesis of these cluster headaches is obscure. The sudden onset, the flushing and the fact that the headaches may be precipitated by histamine injection favors a vascular origin and the significant association with Horner's syndrome suggests a dilatation of the carotid artery within the cranium where the artery is in apposition to the sympathetic plexus. Possibly it is a dilatation within the intra-osseous canal.

SUMMARY

Blackouts (amaurosis fugax) suggest retinal or optic nerve ischemia and commonly result from carotid stenosis or emboli. Photopsia may arise from any portion of the visual system but those produced by vascular lesions in the occiput are usually projected to the contralateral visual field. Especially characteristic are the scintillating scotomas of migraine. Hallucinations may also arise from lesions anywhere in the visual system and are divisible into the highly localizing ictal variety and the non-localizing release variety.

Metamorphopsia indicates macular pathology, while floating opacities indicate particulate matter in the vitreous.

Scotomas are islands of blindness within the visual field, while hemianopias and quadranopias are encroachments onto the midline from the periphery. A central scotoma with loss of vision suggests retinal or optic nerve lesions. Homonymous hemianopia points to a lesion anywhere in the visual system behind the chiasm; bitemporal hemianopia, a lesion of the chiasm itself; binasal hemianopia, a possible lesion of the lateral side of the chiasm or of the optic nerves; and an altitudinal hemianopia, a lesion of the retina or optic nerve.

CHAPTER 5

FUNDUS SIGNS OF SYSTEMIC VASCULAR DISEASE

HYPERTENSION

The minimal ophthalmoscopic manifestation of hypertension is narrowing and irregularity of the retinal arteries (Fig. 62). It begins in the nasal branches but eventually becomes most conspicuous in the temporal branches.

Although the general narrowing and focal constrictions are highly characteristic, they cannot be relied upon as absolute criteria. Nor do they indicate unqualifiedly the degree of hypertension. The chief variable factor is age. Only in the relatively young is the hypertensive narrowing seen in its pure form. In older persons the rigidity of the retinal arteries prevents the narrowing seen in young persons with comparable degrees of hypertension. Evaluation of arteriolar narrowing is thus less reliable in persons of middle age or older.

Over-interpreting arterial narrowing in the fundus is a common failing. When one knows the patient has hypertension, one tends to attach undue significance to questionable changes.

The absolute significance of hypertensive narrowing is also limited by the frequency with which it is seen in conditions other than hypertension. Thus it occurs after arterial occlusion and is particularly severe with abiotrophies (retinitis pigmentosa) that entail loss of the photoreceptors (p. 30). These non-hypertensive conditions, however, show associated abnormalities in the nerve head or clumping of pigment that serve to distinguish them.

Hypertensive narrowing is classically inferred to represent spasm of the arteries.[659] This seems unlikely in view of the diminutive muscularis of the retinal arteries, the absence of any visible changes

74

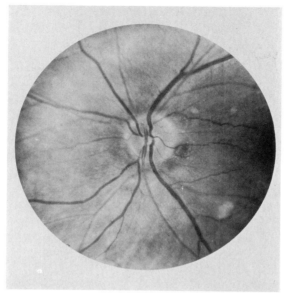

Figure 62   Narrowing and irregularity of the retinal arteries in hypertension.

The patient was a 49 year old man with asymptomatic hypertension (B.P. 220/150). In addition to the arterial narrowing, the fundus shows a cotton-wool opacity in the lower right quadrant and two smaller opacities in the upper quadrant.

in the narrowing over reasonable periods of time, and the histologic evidence of hyalinization. Yet it must be granted that the narrowing is, in young persons at least, completely reversible with measures that lower the blood pressure. This reversibility is less striking in older persons.[433, 525]

When hypertensive retinopathy is combined with internal carotid stenosis and, in consequence, a lower retinal blood pressure in one eye, the hypertensive changes will be less severe on the stenotic side.[325]

Histologic studies of mild hypertension show in cross-sections of the retina mild thickening of the arterial walls and a deposition of additional basement membrane that eventually comprises hyalinization. Trypsin digest preparations have been disappointing in their failure to reveal abnormalities in the vessels that showed the changes ophthalmologically but they have shown a highly characteristic hyalinization and acellularity at the junctions of the precapillary arterioles. This is evident in the increased stainability of these vessels in flat mounts stained by the periodic-acid Schiff method (Fig. 63).

Severe forms of hypertensive retinopathy are characterized not only by marked arterial narrowing but also by hemorrhage, cotton-wool spots, exudate, edema, and papilledema (Fig. 64). The hemorrhages are predominately, but not exclusively, of the flame-shaped va-

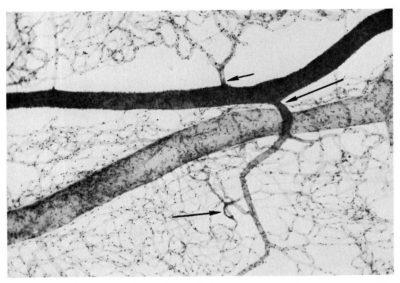

Figure 63 Flat mount of retinal vessels from a patient with hypertension. Characteristic is the increased stainability of the precapillary arterioles (indicated by arrows). (Periodic acid–Schiff stain.)

riety and scattered randomly about the fundus. The cotton-wool spots are often conspicuous and proportional in number to the hemorrhages. They represent infarcts of vessels having the size of precapillary arterioles. The edema produces a gray or "wet" appearance to the entire fundus and shows a correspondingly diffuse leakage by fluoroangiography. Papilledema is a concomitant of severe hypertensive retinopathy, not always correlated with the increased intracranial pressure,[321] and usually connotes an associated hypertensive encephalopathy.[525] By itself it causes an accentuation of the hemorrhages and exudates, especially about the disc, giving rise to a strikingly florid retinopathy.

Despite these severe changes, visual disturbances with hypertensive retinopathy may be surprisingly slight. The degree of functional impairment depends entirely on coincidental involvement of the macula and this is highly variable.

Eclamptic hypertension produces a retinopathy similar to that from other hypertensive causes but the arteriolar narrowing is especially conspicuous, possibly owing to the patient's young age. Frequently a serous detachment of the retina is also present.[663] This latter is characteristically bilateral and involves the lower or dependent parts of the fundi.

Cross-sections of the retina show variably severe hyalinization of the arterial walls with occasional occlusions and recanalizations, cytoid bodies corresponding to the cotton-wool spots, exudate in the

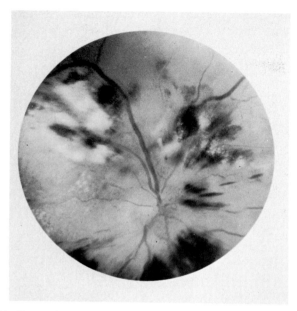

Figure 64   Severe hypertensive retinopathy.

The patient was a 43 year old man with the symptoms of a malignant hypertension (B.P. 220/150). He subsequently died of massive cerebral hemorrhage.

outer reticular and juxtaposed layers, fibrinoid changes in the vessels,[90] cystoid spaces corresponding to the edema, and occasionally serous detachment of the retina. The histologic findings are what one would expect from the ophthalmoscopic appearances. Trypsin digest preparations show in addition widespread occlusion of the arteriolar-venous system.

Many attempts have been made to classify the hypertensive changes into a prognostically useful system. In America the Keith-Wagener classification,[371] dividing the retinopathy into four stages, has been the most popular. The first two stages represent increasingly severe arteriolar changes; the third stage adds hemorrhages and exudate, and the fourth stage adds papilledema. This classification has statistically prognostic value. Yet individual exceptions to it are common and stages 3 and 4 cannot always be accepted as progressive stages of 1 and 2. Thus persons with a hemorrhagic diathesis might, according to this classification, be put in stage 3 because of the hemorrhages, whereas their arteriolar changes and other evidence indicate minimal hypertension. Similarly, patients with mild hypertension but with papilledema due to some other cause (meningiomas or pseudotumor cerebri) have been erroneously classified as stage 4 or malignant hypertension on the basis of their papilledema.[103, 689] It would seem preferable, therefore, to classify hypertensive retinopathy solely on the basis of the arteriolar changes, adding hemorrhages, exudates, and papilledema as additional descriptive features that do not necessarily reflect a progressive stage.

The following system is the author's personal preference: Grade I, mild but definite narrowing and irregularity of lumina in nasal arteries only; Grade II, mild but definite narrowing and irregularity of lumina in temporal as well as the nasal branches; Grade III, moderate to severe narrowing and irregularity of arteries but without obvious occlusion or replacement by white cords; and Grade IV, severe narrowing with replacement of some arteries by white cords. Any stage may be associated with other manifestations of retinopathy and optic neuropathy although the more severe the arterial changes, the more likely are other changes as well.

Hypertensive changes in the choroid are inconspicuous clinically except when they cause retinal detachments but they may be demonstrated angiographically[248] and are obvious histopathologically.[226, 388] In contrast to the uniform hyalinization of hypertensive retinal arteries, the choroidal arteries develop nodular thickenings of their walls and occlusions of the corresponding choriocapillary bed. Serum from these partially obstructed vessels exudes through the pigment epithelium to detach the retina[388] and to produce the pigment irregularities which present clinically as Elschnig spots[183] and pathologically as arterial nodules and secondary pigment epithelial changes.[482]

HYPOTENSION

Systemic hypotension may induce retinal ischemia either on a transient or a permanent basis. The retinal circulation is the first to be affected by a fall in cephalic blood pressure because of the relatively high tissue pressure (about 20 mm Hg) in the eye. Thus blackouts are the common manifestation of vasomotor collapse, as in fainting or shock, and are frequently a presenting symptom in either carotid stenosis or the aortic arch syndrome. They may be precipitated by antihypertensive medication or other blood pressure lowering procedures in persons with impaired circulation.[424] The high intraocular pressure of glaucoma may similarly further jeopardize the circulation in persons with impaired blood flow.[541]

ARTERIOLAR SCLEROSIS

Arteriolar sclerosis of the retinal vessels is, like that of cerebral vessels of a similar size,[2, 460] a process of hyalinization and is not to be confused with atheromatosis (arteriosclerosis) of larger vessels. Nor do the retinal changes reflect what is occurring in the larger vessels having internal elastic lamina and substantial muscular coats.

In contrast to retinal arteries the central artery on the nerve head and the choroidal arteries do have elastic lamina and are capable of developing atheromatosis.

Retinal arteriolar sclerosis consists clinically of a relative opacification of the arterial wall as seen with the ophthalmoscope, an increasing rigidity as inferred from the sinusoidal tortuosity and arteriovenous compression, and a hyalinization as seen histopathologically. It is impossible and probably fruitless to distinguish arteriolar sclerosis from senile arteriopathy.

The opacification of the arterial wall is first evident as a faint obliteration of the underlying venous blood column at an AV crossing (Gunn's sign).[273] Later, ensheathing along the artery and plaque formation at the AV crossing develops (Fig. 65). These opaque mantles are at first mat white but become yellowish and often show scintillating particles as they become lipidized. The fat has been demonstrated histopathologically.[71, 103, 579, 689]

The ensheathing of arteriolar sclerosis is not to be confused with the congenital ensheathing that begins on the nerve head and tapers off in the peripapillary region, nor is it to be confused with the more diffuse ensheathing of the arteries (but more commonly of the veins) that follows papilledema or inflammatory lesions.

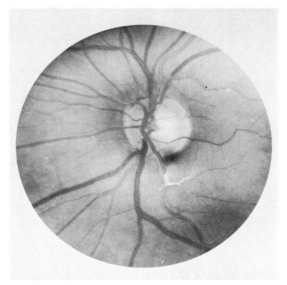

Figure 65 Focal opacification of arterial wall in what is commonly called retinal arteriosclerosis.

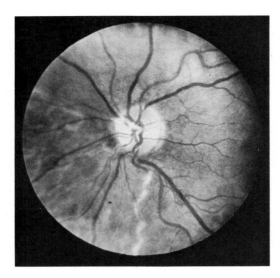

Figure 66 Opaque choroidal vessel running inferiorly from the disc. This is presumed to be a sclerotic choroidal artery.

The rigidity of the senile or sclerotic artery is inferred from the pressure on the vein at the points of AV crossing and the banking of the venous blood (p. 44).

In comparison with sclerosis of the retinal vessels, sclerosis of the choroidal arteries has been poorly documented. Its histopathology more closely resembles that of sclerosis in the rest of the body than that of the retina. White vessels that are often interpreted as arteriosclerosis on clinical grounds are not found to be sclerotic histopathologically.[24] In fact, the vessels are chiefly veins and probably appear white because of the changes in the overlying tissue rather than in the vessels themselves (Fig. 66).[99]

Genuine sclerosis and occlusion of the choroidal arteries are not uncommon and may cause blotchy pigment changes in the periphery but no apparent abnormality in the central fundus. The occlusions may be thrombotic, embolic, or (unlike the retinal arteries) atheromatous. They are often discovered incidentally in eyes post mortem and have been described with polyarteritis,[61, 223, 258, 259, 313] cardiac myxomata,[103, 448, 487, 543, 596] and temporal arteritis.[696]

The pigment clumping may comprise ill-defined zones of chorioretinal "degeneration" similar to that commonly seen in otherwise normal senile eyes or it may occur with white areas that were originally described in nephritis and are called "Elschnig spots,"[183, 388] or the pigmentation may overlie a presumably sclerosed choroidal vessel forming a line that has been likened to a rosary and called Siegrist spot.

DIABETES

Diabetic retinopathy is a prevalent cause of blindness, accounting for from 7 to 20 per cent of all new cases. The frequency depends on the age group and sex.[79] Similar vasculopathies are believed to occur concomitantly in the kidney. The several modern texts[80, 254, 374, 499] devoted exclusively to it and the innumerable papers that deal with it directly and indirectly attest to its importance.

The fundus picture of diabetes comprises three vasopathic types, any one of which tends to predominate for one individual. In order of frequency they are the intraretinal, the proliferative, and the venous types.

The intraretinal type (also termed "background retinopathy") presents ophthalmoscopically as punctate red and white spots in the central fundus (Fig. 67). The red spots are, of course, the hemorrhages and the well-publicized microaneurysms[44] that cannot be easily distinguished from hemorrhages by ophthalmoscopy alone. The white spots are chiefly exudate with usually no more than a few cotton-wool spots.[400] Neither the individual hemorrhages nor the exudate are peculiar to diabetes but their distribution and relative proportions make for the highly characteristic and essentially pathognomonic appearance of diabetic retinopathy.

In the first place, the abnormalities are confined to the posterior portion of the fundus, chiefly to the area bounded by the superior and inferior temporal vessels. The red and especially the white spots tend to occur in clusters or circular zones (Fig. 68). Secondly, the hemorrhages and microaneurysms are predominately punctate because of

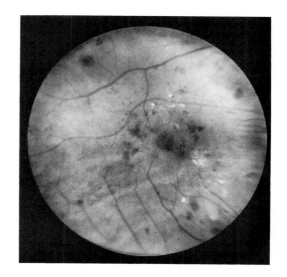

Figure 67 Intraretinal type of diabetic retinopathy. Characteristic are the punctate red spots (hemorrhages and microaneurysms) and white spots (exudate) in the central fundus.

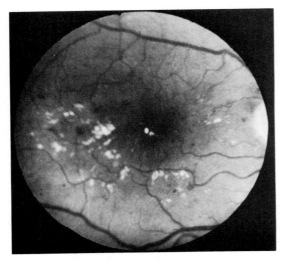

Figure 68 Clusters of exudate in the central fundus of a
diabetic patient.

their deep position in the retina. The flame-shaped hemorrhages that predominate in hypertensive and other vascular retinopathies are relatively inconspicuous in diabetes. The white spots begin as punctate dots but coalesce into sizable conglomerates and occasionally erupt into the subretinal space to form yellowish masses. Some of these form a peculiar circular pattern that is designated circinate retinopathy. Thirdly, a negative but important feature is the absence of gross abnormalities in the major retinal arteries unless there is coexistent hypertension or arteriosclerosis.

The retinopathy is similar regardless of the pathogenesis of the diabetes. In addition to the juvenile and adult onset diabetes, retinopathy occurs with diabetes secondary to pancreatitis, pancreatectomy, hemochromatosis,[270] and Cushing's disease.[474, 580]

Fluoroangiography is of help in detecting early microaneurysms,[9] distinguishing microaneurysms from hemorrhages, and disclosing microaneurysms that were not visible ophthalmoscopically. The microaneurysms then present a striking picture with a predilection for the perimacular area. Fluoroangiography also reveals avascular zones corresponding to the clusters seen ophthalmoscopically surrounded by a corona of microaneurysms and distended capillaries (Fig. 69). Frequently these distended vessels comprise shunts connecting arterioles and venules.[107, 401] When seen ophthalmoscopically without the aid of fluoroangiography, they may be misinterpreted as neovasculogenesis. In fact, they are distended capillaries that have assumed the character of larger vessels.[306]

Although diabetes involves the central area, the fovea itself may be spared so that vision is preserved despite an otherwise extensive

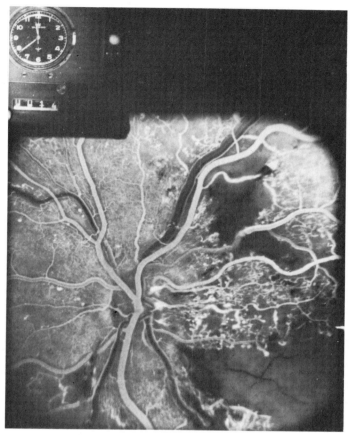

Figure 69 Fluoroangiogram of an eye with moderate diabetic retinopathy. Especially noteworthy are the large avascular areas bordered by microaneurysms and dilated capillaries.

The patient was a 31 year old man who had had diabetes since the age of seven.

retinopathy. Visual acuity is an inadequate guide to the presence or course of diabetic retinopathy.

The proliferative type of diabetic retinopathy (customarily referred to as retinitis proliferans) consists of growth of the retinal vessels into the vitreous (Fig. 70). These vessels derive especially from the disc area[635] where the internal limiting membrane offers the least resistance to their forward extension but they may also arise in the peripheral retina. In the latter case they seem to penetrate the internal limiting membrane at sites where the large retinal vessels are in contact with the internal limiting membrane and in the vicinity of AV crossings.[635] Once these vessels have erupted through the internal limiting membrane, they proliferate floridly either into the vitreous itself or between the vitreous and the retina.[140] Having extended

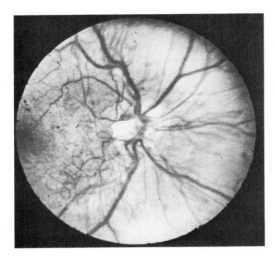

Figure 70 Proliferative type of diabetic retinopathy. Characteristic is the proliferation of vessels arising from the disc area and extending over the adjacent retina.

forward as a plexus of vessels, sometimes in the form of a fan, the vessels then tend to regress while new ones form elsewhere (Fig. 71).[158]

Although the proliferative changes may predominate, some intraretinal retinopathy is practically always present as well. Yet the two do not run parallel and the intraretinal changes are usually less marked with severe proliferative retinopathy.[445] The factors determining the one or other type are obscure but in general the proliferative form occurs more often in young diabetics while the intraretinal form is more characteristic of older diabetics. In either case, however, the retinopathy usually occurs only after one or more decades of diabetes. One survey has indicated, for instance, that whereas retinopathy is

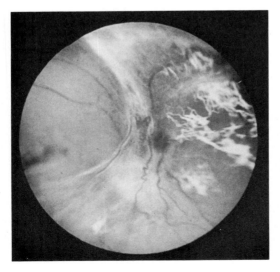

Figure 71 Advanced proliferative retinopathy showing cicatrization and obliteration of some of the vessels. The disc is obscured by the overlying scar tissue.

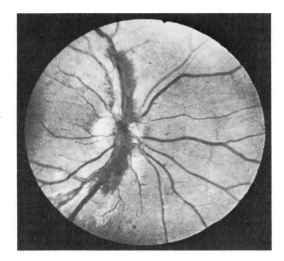

Figure 72   Proliferative retinopathy with hemorrhage from
the vessels over the nerve head.

infrequent in the first 10 years of diabetes, some 90 per cent of patients have it after 30 years and of these, one third are of the proliferative type.[683]

Of the two types, proliferative diabetic retinopathy is the more
serious since it leads to recurrent vitreous hemorrhage (Fig. 72).
These hemorrhages cause precipitous loss of vision and eventuate in a
scar formation that pulls off the retina in a particularly pernicious form
of retinal detachment.

The third and least common type of diabetic retinopathy is that
which affects the larger veins preferentially[362] or exclusively.[603] There
are two venous manifestations which are probably unrelated. The first
is the infrequent engorgement of the large veins (Fig. 73) which come
to have a peculiarly beaded appearance. The pathogenesis of this type
of change is unknown. The second manifestation is venous occlusion.[155] Except for its statistical frequency in diabetes, this occlusion
does not differ from that occurring in non-diabetics and similarly
tends to occur at the lamina cribrosa. It is not necessarily related to the
presence of other types of retinopathy.

The crucial question of a relationship between diabetic retinopathy and systemic control of the diabetes is controversial.[394] Large
series suggest that adequate control has a beneficial effect,[80, 580] but individual cases may show wholly inverse relationships in which gal-
loping retinopathy proceeds despite excellent control or, conversely,
in which minimal retinopathy is present despite poor control. On the
other hand, there does appear to be a positive correlation between the
level of systemic blood pressure and the severity of the diabetic retinopathy.[402]

The histopathology of diabetic retinopathy corroborates many of
the clinical observations and adds important information on the basic

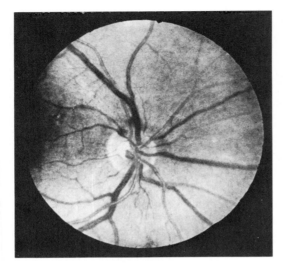

Figure 73 Simple engorgement of retinal veins with diabetes.

The patient was a 40 year old man who, although he had had diabetes since the age of 10, showed no microaneurysms or exudate in his fundi.

pathogenesis of the vasculopathy. Most informative is the study of the intraretinal type in flat mounts of the retinal vasculature prepared by the trypsin digest technique. Microaneurysms constitute the chief feature of these flat mounts. They occur chiefly in the central area, often being massive in and about the macula, and tend to have a cluster distribution about nests of occluded capillaries (Fig. 74). They occur equally in the arteriolar and venular side of the capillary bed, thereby

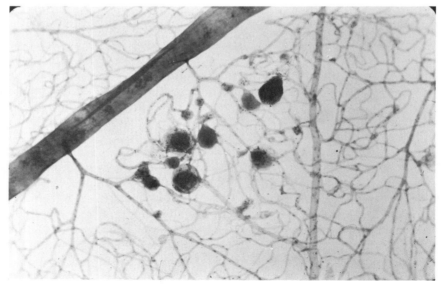

Figure 74 Cluster of microaneurysms surrounding an area of occluded capillaries. (Trypsin digest preparation; PAS-hematoxylin stain.)

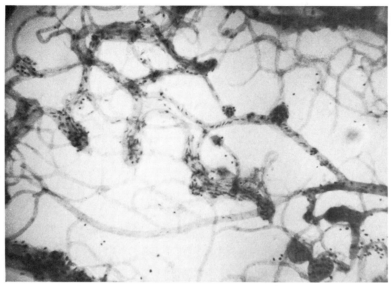

Figure 75 Dilated vessels bordering an area of occluded capillaries. (Trypsin digest preparation; PAS-hematoxylin stain.)

differing from the microaneurysms that follow venous occlusion, which are predominately on the venous side. Just as characteristic as the microaneurysms, however, are the dilated and sinuous capillaries that also border the ischemic clusters (Fig. 75). These eventually form shunts connecting the arterioles and venules (Fig. 76).

The arteriovenous shunts are especially characteristic of diabetes and differ from the arterio-arteriolar shunts that follow arterial occlusions or from the veno-venular shunts that follow venous occlusion.

With the more severe diabetic retinopathy, the ischemic zones coalesce, forming, in advanced cases, large areas of occluded capillaries that are bridged or bordered by a few shunt vessels.

The initial pathology of diabetic retinopathy seems to be loss of the mural cells (intramural pericytes).[98, 111, 445] Whereas the ratio of mural cells to endothelial cells is normally 1:1, it approaches 1:4 in diabetic capillaries.[378, 619, 703] Some capillaries become completely devoid of mural cells while leaving ghostlike mounds at their former sites (Fig. 77). It is reasonable to assume that the loss of these cells which normally provide tone to the capillaries allows the dilation of the capillary wall locally in the form of a microaneurysm or diffusely in the form of an oversized capillary. It is also reasonable to assume that these enlarged vessels will dry up the adjacent capillaries, accounting for the clusters of ischemia. On the other hand, arguments have been advanced suggesting that the ischemia is primary.[90, 401]

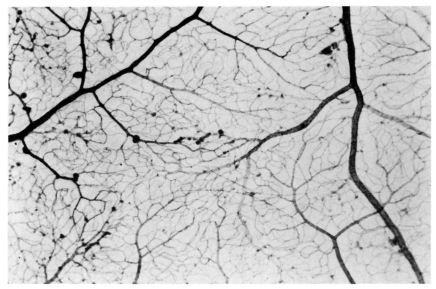

Figure 76   Panoramic view of retinal vessels, showing a shunt vessel connecting an arteriole (on the left) with a venule (on the right). Also noteworthy are the microaneurysms, the dilated capillaries, and the large area of occluded capillaries. (Trypsin digest preparation; PAS-hematoxylin stain.)

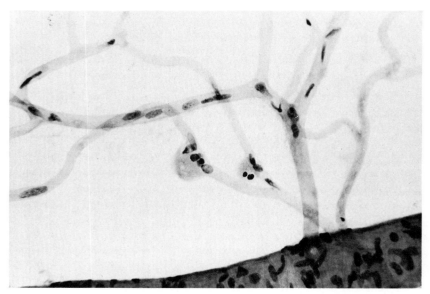

Figure 77   Capillaries from an eye with diabetic retinopathy showing loss of mural cells and proliferation of endothelial cells (especially in the region of a microaneurysm).

The distension of the vessel wall, in the form of microaneurysms or of diffuse enlargements, results in a sequence of events that may be illustrated by the life cycle of the microaneurysm. At first the aneurysm has a thin wall with nothing but a tenuous basement membrane and endothelial lining. As the wall becomes stretched, the endothelium proliferates and lays down new basement membrane (possibly as a protective mechanism). Repetition of this process produces an onion-skin nodule in which basement membrane and entrapped endothelial cells form a nodule. For some time the aneurysm has a recognizable lumen and patent connection with the capillary but further deposition of basement membrane results ultimately in total occlusion of the aneurysm. The entrapped endothelial cells disintegrate to leave a hyalinized nodule which stains intensely by the periodic acid-Schiff method and eventually becomes, like most pathologic hyaline membranes, sudanophilic.

Flat mounts stained by the periodic acid-Schiff method do not show the diffuse increase in basement membrane that has been postulated to underly diabetic vasculopathy elsewhere.[602] However, the microaneurysms and the diffusely distended capillaries do show focally increased basement membrane which has been thought to be the counterpart of the hyaline nodules in the Kimmelstiel-Wilson kidneys.[221]

Microaneurysms similar to those in the retina have not been found by standard microscopy in the brain or other tissues[21, 222] but no comprehensive search of extraretinal vessels has been reported using modern methods of whole mount preparations.

It is paradoxic that those thin-walled aneurysms which, being filled with blood, were the most obvious by ordinary ophthalmoscopy and fluoroangiography are the least conspicuous in flat mounts and that the occluded and hyalinized aneurysms which stand out so strikingly in flat mounts are not visible clinically. Except for these seemingly paradoxic but logical differences the flat mounts show a good correlation with the fluoroangiographic findings.[147, 399]

The later and final stages in the aneurysmal decline are characterized by disintegration and phagocytosis of the basement membrane and of the hematogenous products that have leaked out of the aneurysm.

This somewhat simplified overview of the rise and fall of a microaneurysm has not taken into account other suggestions for its pathogenesis. Mention should be made of the proposals that microaneurysms result from stasis in veins with degeneration of endothelium,[42, 45] neovascular buds,[25, 49, 687] traction phenomena,[692, 693] herniation of wall at sites of lipid deposits,[530] lipid thrombi with secondary ischemia,[90] and primary defects in the basement membrane.[10]

Cross-sectional microscopy of eyes with diabetic retinopathy has been less informative than flat mounts but it does provide significant additional information. The hemorrhages in the retina are apt to be abundant and are especially prone to be deep. They frequently erupt through the posterior surface and form subretinal hemorrhages with eventual replacement by lipid metamorphosis. In no other condition, except Coats' disease, is there such a conspicuous lipid phagocytosis in the subretinal and outer retinal layers.

In contrast to the intraretinal type of diabetic retinopathy, that of the proliferative type is best studied in cross-sectional preparations. The vascular sprouts coming from the disc or retina have a well-developed endothelium but only abortive basement membrane. They are, however, accompanied by a fibroglial stroma that may at first be cellular but eventually converts into a diaphanous, acellular tissue with only skeletal remnants of the vascular channels. This constitutes the veil, seen ophthalmoscopically, that replaces the proliferating vessels.

The pathogenesis of this proliferative type is obscure. It may represent a bypass for venous occlusion but, if so, its predilection for diabetes and not for the common tributary occlusions is unexplained. The site of eruption overlying a point where the major vessels are in contact with the internal limiting membrane seems to represent a vulnerable spot since rupture at these sites is a common histologic finding in otherwise normal eyes. The vessels which grow into the vitreous are similar to those of granulation tissue with large channels, leaky walls, and absence of mural cells. They do not form microaneurysms.

Studies on diabetic retinopathy have been hampered by the lack of a good animal model. Although diabetes occurs spontaneously in many animals, especially well documented in the dog,[185] and can be produced experimentally by alloxan or corticosteroids, it has not shown the retinopathy comparable to that of human beings. Even the monkey, which has a central fundus and a vascular architecture like that of man, has shown only an abortive retinopathy.[184, 245] Most other laboratory animals have been equally disappointing.[642] The early reports of retinal microaneurysms in rabbits induced by alloxan[208] and by corticoids[48] have not been confirmed.

The dog provides, perhaps, the best model, for typical microaneurysms, though few in number, have been repeatedly observed.[185, 244, 513, 515, 591] They occur with spontaneous or induced diabetes but only after the diabetes has been present for from two to four years.[185] Its severity seems to relate to the level of hyperglycemia and to be benefited by adequate control of the diabetes.[184]

Treatment of diabetic retinopathy continues in the cycle of trials and errors, hopes and frustrations. The retinopathy is not clearly benefited by control of the diabetes.[394] Diet is not known to be preventive. Pituitary ablation first introduced as the result of a fortuitous cure in a patient with pituitary necrosis[531] has been induced by surgical resection, stalk section, radiation, and cryotherapy. The initial benefit

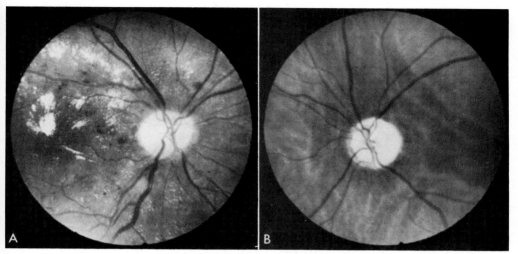

Figure 78 The two eyes of a patient with diabetic retinopathy, illustrating the effect of prior vascular occlusive disease. The right eye *(A)* shows typical diabetic retinopathy but the left eye *(B)*, which had previously had an occlusion of the central retinal artery, shows none of the abnormalities of diabetic retinopathy.

is often dramatic but the late results have been less encouraging.[446] The procedure has now been largely discontinued.[499] A host of drugs have been recommended and eventually discarded. Aldose reductase inhibitors seem to hold some promise for the future.[353, 582] In the meantime photocoagulation is widely used to obliterate the leaking or proliferating vessels by means of the xenon arc or ruby and argon lasers.[70, 348, 423, 427, 469, 498, 514, 634, 681]

In general it may be said that anything which obliterates the capillaries will prevent diabetic retinopathy. Thus eyes with high myopia or those with antecedent occlusive vascular disease will not develop diabetic retinopathy as readily as do the previously normal eyes (Fig. 78).[240] This is the rationale for inducing a mild but widespread retinopathy prophylactically.[50, 468] By contrast, anything which increases the retinal vascular pressure over the intraocular pressure will increase the diabetic retinopathy.[168] Thus systemic hypertension or ocular hypotension will have an adverse effect whereas systemic hypotension or ocular hypertension (glaucoma) will have a salutary effect.[240]

ANEMIA

The retinopathy which occurs with severe anemia is characterized by hemorrhages, cotton-wool spots, and occasionally papilledema (Fig. 79). There is nothing about these retinal signs which alone

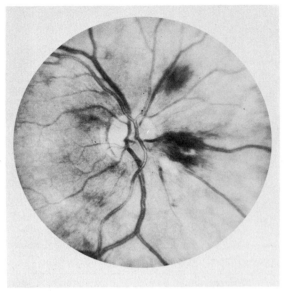

Figure 79 Anemic retinopathy with hemorrhages and cotton-wool spots but normal vessels.

The patient was a 40 year old woman who had a megaloblastic anemia secondary to folic acid deficiency. Hematocrit was 6 per cent.

points to the diagnosis. The hemorrhages are either flame-shaped or blotchy, 1/4 to 1 disc diameter in size, and not punctate. They occasionally have white centers and are then called Roth spots (p. 52). The cotton-wool spots may be single but are not otherwise atypical. The papilledema is nonspecific and its pathogenesis is obscure, but it resolves with correction of the anemia.[393, 645] Perhaps the most suggestive aspect of the fundus picture is the normality of the vessels despite other evidence of vascular retinopathy.

The pathogenesis of the retinopathy is far from clear. While the hemorrhages usually occur with hemoglobin levels that are less than 50 per cent of normal,[46, 369, 454, 465] they may be absent even when the anemia is much worse than this. Probably other factors, such as thrombocytopenia,[393, 465, 556] hypoxic damage to the vessel wall,[393, 655] and age,[465] are contributory. Children rarely develop a retinopathy despite severe anemia.

Vision may or may not be impaired with the retinopathy of anemia. Occasionally the visual loss simulates a bilateral retrobulbar neuritis and may culminate in optic atrophy.[180] Acute blood loss, occurring most commonly with gastrointestinal hemorrhage, produces a visual loss that usually comes on several days after the hemorrhagic event. It, too, is associated with retinal hemorrhages, cotton-wool spots, and visual loss. It is no doubt ischemic in origin, showing the expected histologic changes,[32] and may end in blindness with optic atrophy (see Fig. 56, p. 62) but may, contrariwise, show remarkable recovery. Many cases of anemic retinopathy are asymptomatic and discovered only on routine ophthalmoscopy.[510]

COLLAGENOSES

That group of diseases which for the present are incorporated under the omnibus term collagenoses frequently show a vascular type of retinopathy. Retinal changes have been noted in lupus erythematosus, scleroderma, dermatomyositis,[72, 162] polyarteritis (p. 104), and rheumatoid arthritis.

The retinopathy is often compounded by hypertensive features which, in disseminated lupus erythematosus particularly, coexist. In the absence of hypertension, the prime fundus abnormality consists of cotton-wool spots (Fig. 80). These are more numerous than the number of hemorrhages would lead one to expect and at times are the sole abnormality (Fig. 81). The fundus picture suggests a micro-arteriolar as opposed to a venular process, an interpretation that is consistent with the histopathologic changes.[34] The waxing and waning of the cotton-wool spots have been plotted in a typical case of lupus erythematosus over a period of one year until the eventual demise of the patient and demonstration of cytoid bodies in the retina.[67]

With adequate treatment of the collagenoses, usually by steroids, the spots may disappear, leaving an entirely normal fundus.

Polyarteritis presents a special subgroup of the collagenoses not only because of the occasional occlusion of the central artery in this disease[55, 190] but more especially because of the frequency with which the choroid is involved, as shown by clinical[62] and histopathologic[61, 223, 258, 259, 313] evidence, with consequent detachment of the retina.

HYPERLIPEMIA AND HYPERCHOLESTEREMIA

Elevated blood lipids may produce distinctive fundus appearances. The lactescence from increased neutral triglycerides is indicated by a characteristically white or pale appearance of the retinal vessels (Fig. 82) and occasionally by a pallor of the entire fundus. It becomes evident as the lipid level exceeds 2.5 per cent[657] and occurs nonspecifically with hyperlipemia of diabetes, alcoholic cirrhosis of the liver, or hypopituitary myxedema,[633] or may be of genetic origin. It produces no recognized functional disturbance in the eye and is completely reversible once the blood lipids return to near normal levels.

Hypercholesteremia (in contrast to hypertriglyceridemia) may in-

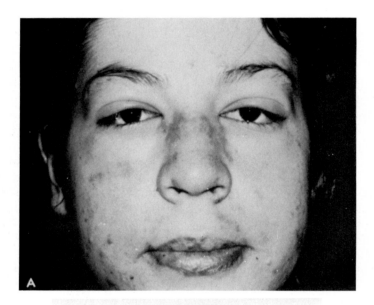

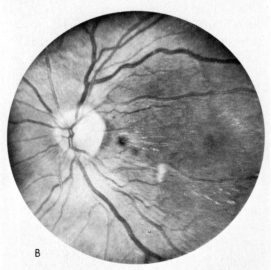

Figure 80 Butterfly rash (A) and solitary cotton-wool spot (B) in a patient with lupus erythematosus.

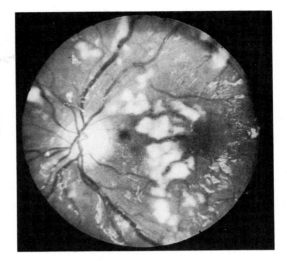

Figure 81 Multiple cotton-wool spots in a patient with dermatomyositis.

duce characteristic white deposits along retinal arteries, forming a string of beads appearance (Fig. 83). This is an infrequent occurrence (apparently not previously reported) and requires a cholesterol level in the range of 400 mg per 100 ml or higher.* Vision will be affected only if there is associated arterial occlusion. The deposits may disappear with lowering of the blood cholesterol level. They have not, as yet, been examined pathologically.

─────────────

*Of the author's five patients, all were in excess of this except one whose cholesterol level was never higher than 350 mg per 100 ml.

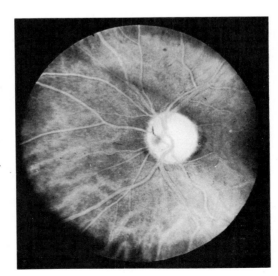

Figure 82 Lactescence of the retinal vessels in hyperlipemia.

The patient was a 40 year old man who was found, on a routine screening test, to have a neutral fat level in his blood of 1078 mg per 100 ml. He was an alcoholic with suspected cirrhosis of the liver.

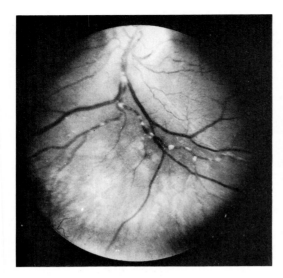

Figure 83 Beading of the retinal artery in a patient with hypercholesteremia.

The patient was a 37 year old man with a serum cholesterol level of 400 mg per 100 ml.

ANGIOID STREAKS

Angioid streaks consist of branching lines with a superficial resemblance to vessels (Fig. 84). They are at first brown but later are replaced by a mixture of white scar tissue and black pigment. Most characteristic is the pattern that these lines take: one incomplete circle surrounds the disc and is connected with coarse radiating lines that extend toward the periphery in octopus fashion. Many variations of this pattern are encountered and occasionally the lines appear to be randomly distributed. In all cases, however, they are maximal in the posterior part of the eye and predominate about the disc.

A less familiar but nonetheless characteristic fundus abnormality in eyes with angioid streaks is an area of speckled pigmentation[58, 247, 588] or peau d'orange appearance. This, which has been called a forme fruste of the entity, is ill defined and usually temporal to the macula.

Angioid streaks are present for years without giving rise to symptoms but they are prone to cause hemorrhage, especially as the result of blunt trauma.[550] Hemorrhage is especially common in the submacular area with resultant severe loss of vision. The blood is eventually replaced by connective tissue and metaplastic pigment epithelium to produce the ophthalmoscopic picture of disciform macular degeneration.

Fluoroangiography shows in the early stages an increased transmission of the choroidal fluorescence in the region of the streaks. In the more advanced stages the fluorescein is taken up by the scar tissue as a persistent stain.[550, 608]

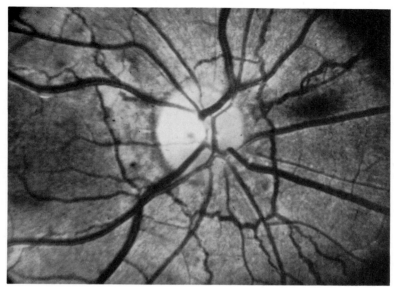

Figure 84 Angioid streaks. Noteworthy is the general arrangement of an incomplete circle about the disc with lines radiating from this toward the periphery.

The systemic condition most frequently associated with angioid streaks is pseudoxanthoma elasticum in the entity known as the Grönblad-Strandberg syndrome.[509] Approximately one half of all cases of angioid streaks show this association.[119, 509, 573] Pseudoxanthoma elasticum is an elastodystrophy of the skin affecting primarily the crease areas (for example, nape of the neck, axilla, and antecubital regions). It presents clinically a yellowish, leathery texture that is easily recognized. Histologically, pseudoxanthoma elasticum shows proliferation and fragmentation of elastic tissue in the deep dermis. It is called elastic tissue because it takes elastic stains but it differs from normal elastic fibers in its deeper position, its curlicue fragments, and its calcifo-siderosis.

Pseudoxanthoma elasticum consists of the same histopathologic particles that constitute pinguecula of the conjunctiva, but as far as is known, there is no clinical association of the two, nor is there any definite association of pseudoxanthoma elasticum with senile elastosis of the skin.[509]

Other systemic conditions associated with angioid streaks are Paget's disease (approximately 10 per cent of patients with advanced Paget's disease have angioid streaks) and a miscellany of cardiovascular abnormalities that are manifest clinically in hypertension, intermittent claudication, and gastrointestinal hemorrhage and pathologically by calcification of the walls of medium-sized arteries. An

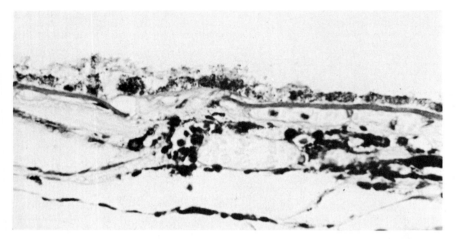

Figure 85 Rupture of a calcified Bruch's membrane with pigmentary changes and extension of choroidal tissue through the rupture.

The patient was a 65 year old woman with pseudoxanthoma elasticum, Paget's disease, and angioid streaks.

association has also been claimed in sickle cell disease,[243, 505] Ehlers-Danlos syndrome,[267] lead poisoning,[146] and acromegaly.[340, 508, 700]

The histologic abnormalities in angioid streaks have been well documented. The essential abnormality is an unusual brittleness of Bruch's membrane.[383] With angioid streaks this membrane becomes prematurely basophilic through deposition of calcium and iron[278, 652] and is prone to rupture along lines of mechanical stress.[3] The initial streaks seen ophthalmoscopically are the sites of rupture and represent separation of the edges of Bruch's membrane and its attached pigment epithelium (Fig. 85). With involvement of the choriocapillaris in this rupture, hemorrhage occurs into the subretinal space. Eventually blood vessels grow through the rupture to cause further leakage and hemorrhage. These then are replaced by fibroplastic tissue which accounts for the late ophthalmoscopic picture of advanced angioid streaks. The severe visual loss is due to the preferential localization of this process for the central fundus. While there is no obvious explanation for this central localization, it is the same process that underlies disciform degeneration unassociated with angioid streaks.

The cause of angioid streaks is obscure but some cases seem to follow an autosomal recessive transmission. The association with pseudoxanthoma elasticum and with calcification of arteries suggests a disease of elastic tissue. The association with Paget's disease, sickle cell disease, and acromegaly is less readily explained.

Treatment of angioid streaks is generally ineffectual although leaks that are spotted by fluoroangiography may be sealed by photocoagulation to forestall subretinal hemorrhages.

MISCELLANEOUS VASCULOPATHIES

Retinal hemorrhages and other types of retinopathy are surprisingly infrequent with purpuric diseases (hemophilia, thrombocytopenia) and with anticoagulant medication unless anemia[556] or local vasculopathy is also present.

Leukemia may be accompanied by severe hemorrhagic retinopathy with obstruction of the small vessels and capillaries. The distended veins have a linked sausage appearance.[7] Flat mounts of the retinal vessels from persons dying of leukemia illustrate the hemodynamic problems (Fig. 86). Extravasation of leukemic cells out of these vessels may result in local tumor formation[412] and is not necessarily related to the white count in the blood.[64]

Thrombotic thrombocytopenia is especially apt to cause a serous extravasation from the choriocapillaris and, in consequence, a detachment of the retina which, like that due to other systemic diseases, is usually bilateral and potentially reversible.

Coats' disease and the telangiectasia of Leber are retinal vasculo-

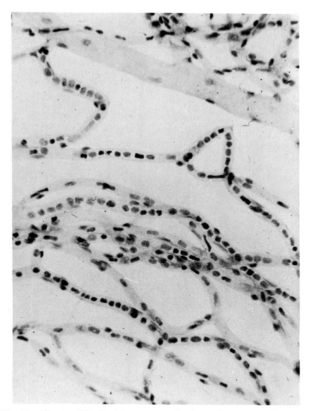

Figure 86 Capillaries filled with tumor cells from the retina of a person who died of leukemia. (Trypsin digest preparation; PAS-hematoxylin stain.)

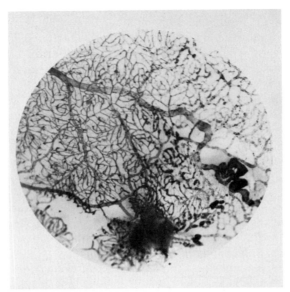

Figure 87   Telangiectatic vessels from the peripheral retina of a patient with Coats' disease. (Trypsin digest preparation; PAS-hematoxylin stain.)

pathies occurring usually in young males and limited to one eye.[315] Typically, Coats' disease consists of telangiectases of the peripheral vessels (Fig. 87) and local hemorrhages in and beneath the retina. Leber's telangiectases differ in involving the more central vessels. The hemorrhages, together with the serum, undergo a lipid metamorphosis that gives the characteristic ophthalmoscopic picture of a yellowish scintillating mass beneath the retina. This may be mistaken for tumor. Histologically the telangiectatic vessels show profuse basement membrane proliferation[540] within the retina and massive lipid phagocytosis beneath the retina. The pathogenesis of Coats' disease is unknown but it appears to be a local process without systemic correlates. Some observers believe the primary fault is in the endothelium and that the telangiectases are secondary.[644]

As noted elsewhere (p. 44), multiple sclerosis is sometimes associated with ensheathing of the retinal veins. "Spasms" of the retinal artery have also been described during the scotoma phase of multiple sclerosis.[66] This surprising observation would be highly significant if it were confirmed.

SUMMARY

The principle ophthalmoscopic signs of hypertension are narrowing of the arteries and irregularity of the arterial lumina. These are most distinctive and reliable in young persons. Hemorrhages and papilledema may be secondary to some cause other than hypertension and are therefore not reliable indices in themselves. Severe hypertensive retinopathy is, nevertheless, associated with diffuse hemorrhages, exudate, cotton-wool spots, and papilledema. Histologically, the arteries show hyaline occlusion of their walls and an especially characteristic increased stainability of the precapillary arterioles.

Retinal arterial hypotension produces retinal ischemia and blackouts. These occur with fainting but are especially prominent in carotid stenosis or the aortic arch syndrome.

What is called arteriolar sclerosis is an increased rigidity of the retinal arteries of older persons manifest by tortuosity of the arteries, opacification of their walls, and arteriovenous compression. It is not comparable to the arteriosclerosis and atheromatosis of arteries containing elastic laminae.

Intraretinal or background retinopathy comprises the most frequent form of diabetic retinopathy. It is marked primarily by punctate red spots, consisting of hemorrhages and microaneurysms, and by yellowish white, often confluent dots made up of exudate. Together they occupy chiefly the posterior regions of the fundus. Vascular proliferative retinopathy is also a frequent form of diabetic retinopathy and is far more serious since the repeated intravitreal hemorrhages often lead to irrevocable blindness. Dilation and congestion of the retinal veins is a third type of diabetic retinopathy with or without venous occlusion.

The pathogenesis of intraretinal diabetic retinopathy appears to depend on preferential loss of the mural cells and consequent bulging of the capillary walls in the form of leaky microaneurysms and dilation of capillaries in the form of shunt vessels. With proliferative retinopathy, vessels erupt into the vitreous through the internal limiting membrane but the pathogenesis of this neovasculogenesis is not readily explained.

Anemia may present a nonspecific retinopathy consisting of hemorrhages, cotton-wool spots, and papilledema, with or without loss of vision. The collagenoses, uncomplicated by hypertension, may also show a vascular retinopathy but tend to have a predominance of cotton-wool spots rather than hemorrhages. Hyperlipemia produces a characteristic lactescence of the retinal vessels without any functional impairment whereas hypercholesteremia produces either no visible abnormality or, in rare cases, white deposits along the arteries.

Angioid streaks are circumpapillary and form radial lines in the fundus that present branching patterns suggestive of vessels but which are in actuality ruptures of Bruch's membrane. Angioid streaks have been reported with many conditions but are particularly associated with pseudoxanthoma elasticum of the skin and with Paget's disease.

Other vasculopathies in the fundus are those of leukemia with local tumor formation, thrombotic thrombocytopenia with detachment of the retina, and the telangiectases of Coats and Leber.

CHAPTER 6

OCCLUSIVE ARTERIAL DISEASE IN THE EYE

PRIMARY

Retina

Occlusion of the central retinal artery produces unmistakable signs and symptoms. The patient, who may previously have had transient episodes of blurred vision, develops sudden blindness in one eye. The blindness may be complete, but perception of hand movements may be preserved in that portion of the visual field corresponding to the cilioretinal artery. A mild ache in the eye may be present but severe pain suggests involvement of the ophthalmic artery as well.

By the time the patient reports for examination the circulation is often restored but if complete occlusion has lasted more than 20 minutes, the blindness is generally irreversible. Ophthalmoscopy within the first hour or so reveals surprisingly little. The eye is unquestionably blind, as indicated by the failure of the pupil to react to light, but the disc shows typically no more than mild pallor and the arteries are only mildly attenuated. In the unusual event that the occlusion has persisted to the time of examination, the arteries may be very narrow and the vein will show boxcar segmentation. In the presence of a slow but not arrested circulation, segmentation may be brought out by gentle pressure on the globe during ophthalmoscopy. A more subtle sign of partial obstruction of the central artery is evident in the type of collapse induced in the artery with pressure on the globe. Instead of demonstrating the crisp pulsation which occurs normally when the intraocular pressure exceeds the retinal diastolic pressure, the obstructed artery will merely collapse and show a comparatively slow refill as the pressure is removed.

102

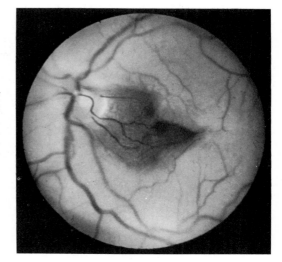

Figure 88 Opacification of the retina following transient occlusion of the central retinal artery but sparing the region corresponding to an area supplied by two cilioretinal arteries.

If the obstruction of the central retinal artery is secondary to occlusion of the ophthalmic artery, the intraocular pressure will be pathologically low (that is, in the range of 4 to 6 mm Hg instead of 20 mm Hg).[69]

The opacification of the retina and the central cherry red spot, which are the classic signs of central retinal artery occlusion, become apparent only after several hours and persist for two or more weeks (Fig. 88). The opacity is most dense about the fovea and fades progressively toward the periphery. It disappears as the ganglion cells disintegrate and as the optic nerve becomes atrophic. Hemorrhages are not a feature of central retinal artery occlusion unless the vein is also obstructed.

The larger retinal vessels may remain ophthalmoscopically normal indefinitely or they may become white threads (Fig. 89).[439] Sometimes they eventually develop lipid deposits in their walls and then present a yellowish scintillating opacification. This opacification may either increase or decrease with time.

Ancillary tests to confirm the diagnosis are interesting but usually unnecessary. Prompt fluoroangiography will reveal either a retardation or a complete failure in filling of the vessels depending on the degree of obstruction.[237] Electroretinographic responses show minimal or transient abnormality as long as only the central retinal artery is affected[305, 352, 367] but will be extinguished if the ophthalmic artery, and thereby the choroidal arteries, are obstructed as well.[85]

The usual site for central retinal artery obstruction is the lamina cribrosa where the periarterial fibrous membrane presents a mechanical barrier to expansion of the artery. Atheromata and emboli are the two principal causes of obstruction. The two are difficult to differentiate in the older age group because the lamina cribrosa is not visible

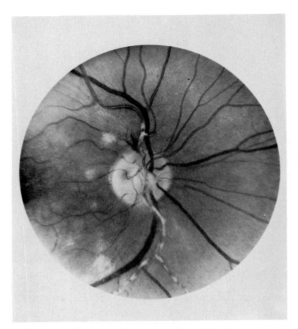

Figure 89   Opacification of the arterial wall following occlusion.

clinically but emboli are always suspect in younger persons, especially when there is associated evidence of rheumatic heart disease, cardiac myxomata, or mucor infection. Atheromatosis may produce progressive stenosis or a precipitous occlusion with hemorrhage beneath an atheromatous plaque.[130] Other causes of central retinal artery occlusion are carotid stenosis (p. 111), vasculitis (p. 136), polyarteritis,[55, 190, 666] collagenoses (p. 93), giant cell arteritis (p. 132), and a high ratio of the intraocular pressure to the retinal blood pressure. Thus artery occlusion may occur hydrostatically with either the high intraocular pressure of glaucoma[249, 707] or the low retinal blood pressure of carotid stenosis[144] or the aortic arch syndrome (p. 113).

While the processes that obstruct the central retinal artery may spare the cilioretinal artery, the reverse also occurs wherein the cilioretinal artery is obstructed, producing a paracentral scotoma, without involvement of the central retinal artery (Fig. 90).

Branch retinal artery occlusion simulates that of the central retinal artery except that it involves only one sector (most commonly the temporal branches; Fig. 91). It also provides a more accessible view for study of the pathogenetic process and for an evaluation of the collateral circulation.[652] A few splinter hemorrhages may border the infarcted area but they are not a conspicuous feature. Central vision is usually spared and the patient may be unaware of the field defect.

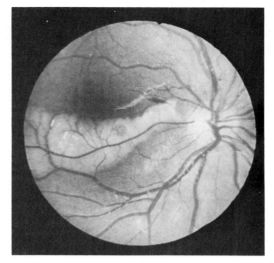

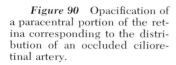 Opacification of a paracentral portion of the retina corresponding to the distribution of an occluded cilioretinal artery.

The feathery white areas above and below the opacity are highlights reflected from the surface of the retina.

Branch occlusion is usually caused by emboli. These emboli may be calcific or lipidic and often lodge at the bifurcation of an artery. Branch occlusions also occur secondary to local inflammations in the eye, as well as in the collagenoses, sickle cell disease, and Eales' disease (p. 116).

The histopathology of retinal artery occlusion is characterized by the loss of all the inner glioneuronal layers of the retina down to and including part of the bipolar cell layers (Fig. 92). This latter layer is the divide between the retinal and choroidal blood supply.

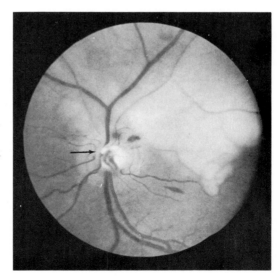

Figure 91 Occlusion of the superior temporal artery. Noteworthy is the embolus on the disc (indicated by arrow) and a hemorrhage at the lower edge of the opaque retina.

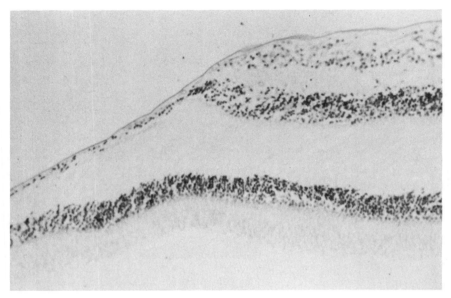

Figure 92 Cross-section of the retina near the macula showing an infarcted area (on the left) and normal area (on the right). The infarction had caused disappearance of all the inner layers of the retina.

The patient had had an occlusion of the central retinal artery but sparing of the cilioretinal artery. The cross-section was prepared at the junction of the two.

The remarkable feature is the nearly total disappearance of the tissue so that the inner limiting membrane comes almost into contact with the residual bipolar cells without appreciable gliosis or other cellular reaction. Flat mounts prepared by trypsin digestion show varying degrees of hyalinization of these arteries and extensive acellularity of the capillary bed, while cross-sections show recanalization.[366]

Experimental occlusion of the central retinal artery in the monkey has shown fluoroangiographic and pathologic changes similar to those in man.[408]

Treatment of retinal artery occlusion has been discouraging. No drugs have withstood the test of time despite enthusiastic protagonists, and some of the recommended drugs may have had an adverse effect.[224] There is logic in giving CO_2 since this dilates the retinal vessels; this together with ocular massage has been reported to have a beneficial effect.[288] Paracentesis is rarely successful.[598]

Anticoagulants and endarterectomy are reasonable for threatened occlusion, as suggested by periodic blackouts. The problem in evaluating their efficacy is to know which cases would have gone on to permanent occlusion. However, success has been reported with partial occlusion even when treatment has been begun hours after the onset of amaurosis.

The prognosis for recovery of vision is poor but in some cases in which the obstruction has been incomplete and especially in which the macula is supplied by both a cilioretinal and retinal artery considerable recovery may be a pleasant surprise. On the other hand, most patients not only remain blind but some (estimated at 5 per cent)[366] develop the enigmatic neovascularization of the iris and attendant hemorrhagic glaucoma (p. 127).[432, 522, 527, 605]

Loss of vision from central retinal artery occlusion is such a major calamity that one tends to equate it with the major strokes of intracranial origin. One must remember, however, that the arteries involved are of an entirely different order of magnitude. With the possible exception of the internal capsule region, vascular occlusions in the brain, comparable in size to those in the eye, would produce little if any overt symptoms. Such minute infarcts in the cortex are frequently found post mortem in the brains of persons who had given no history of functional impairment during life.

Another significant difference between vascular accidents in the retina and those in the brain is the relative irreversibility of the former. The blindness from retinal artery occlusion is permanent if the occlusion has persisted for 20 minutes or so, whereas the blindness (or hemianopia) of cerebral origin may progressively improve for weeks after the accident.

Optic Nerve

Occlusion of the short ciliary arteries that supply the optic nerve head comprises an entity that is variously called ischemic optic neuropathy, vascular optic neuritis, and opticomalacia. The common causes are atheromatosis and temporal arteritis (p. 132) but it has also been reported with polyarteritis.[260]

Ischemic optic neuropathy presents with total or partial blindness (often an altitudinal hemianopia), swelling of the disc with a few peripapillary hemorrhages, and frequently a curious combination of pallor of one portion of the disc and simultaneous dilatation of the capillaries in another portion (Fig. 93). The retinal arteries may be narrow but the retina does not show the opacity or cherry red spot that is characteristic of retinal artery occlusion. The second eye is apt to develop a similar ischemic neuropathy some months or years after the first eye, thus culminating in the tragedy of total blindness. The onset is dramatically sudden in most cases but on occasion it may be gradual.[396]

Differentiation from an inflammatory optic neuritis offers a problem that is sometimes insoluble. Both show swelling of the disc, dilatation of the papillary vessels, and gross leakage by fluoroangiography. The absence of pain, however, and the early pallor of the disc favor the diagnosis of ischemia. A central scotoma may suggest an optic neuritis whereas an altitudinal hemianopia suggests a vascular optic neuropathy but even these are, at times, interchangeable.

Temporal arteritis produces the typical picture of ischemic optic neuropathy but differs from the atheromatous type in the elevated sedimentation

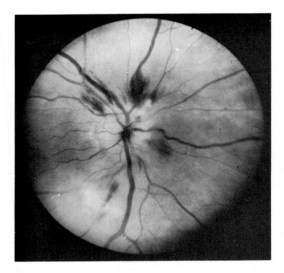

Figure 93 Ischemic optic neuropathy. The typical ophthalmoscopic abnormalities are swelling of the disc and peripapillary hemorrhages associated with sudden blindness, but there are no abnormalities of the retinal vessels and no opacification of the retina.

rate and tenderness along the temporal arteries. Moreover, the second eye in temporal arteritis tends to become involved within 1 to 3 weeks instead of months to years as with atheromatosis.

The optic neuropathy of diabetes may have a vascular basis but it has not been well studied. Alternative suggestions are that it represents either a diabetic neuritis (which seems likely for the childhood type[621]) or a form of tobacco neuritis.[51, 628, 639] The optic neuropathy of pernicious anemia has been similarly interpreted as a form of tobacco neuritis.[211]

A few pathologic specimens which have become available for study in the early stages of ischemic optic neuropathy have shown swelling of the nerve head anterior to the lamina cribrosa and replacement of the nerve substance posterior to the lamina by lipid macrophages (typical gitter cell reaction).[396] Late cases of ischemic optic neuropathy show the expected loss of nerve substance (Fig. 94).[100, 129] The occlusive changes in the ciliary arteries have been documented only in the case of temporal arteritis.[310, 449, 620]

Ischemic optic neuropathy has been induced in monkey eyes by cauterization of the posterior ciliary arteries.[301] The clinical and histopathologic changes were similar to those occurring in human eyes with ischemic optic neuropathy.

The treatment of ischemic optic neuropathy of arteriosclerotic origin is the same as that for occlusive disease elsewhere and is similarly ineffectual once the condition has been established. Nevertheless, antecedent blackouts should be treated with long-term anticoagulants in the hope that collateral circulation will develop to bypass the occluded ciliary arteries.

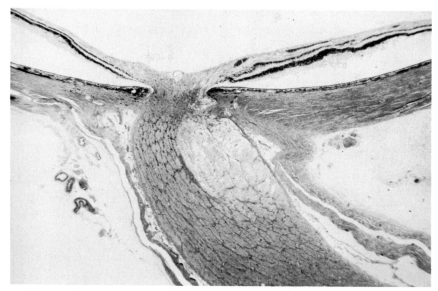

Figure 94 Ischemic optic neuropathy characterized by extensive loss of optic nerve structures behind the lamina cribrosa.

The patient was a 72 year old woman with a history of hypertension (B.P. 210/100) and mild diabetes. She died of coronary occlusion and overwhelming sepsis. She had not volunteered any visual symptoms in her terminal illness and ophthalmoscopy had not been done.

Choroid

Because of its inaccessibility for clinical examination and more particularly because of its rich anastomoses, occlusion of the choroidal arteries has received little attention from clinicians. It does appear, however, that the large areas of pigment mottling in the periphery of the retina, including possibly pavement degeneration and Elschnig spots, and possibly some of the pigmentary changes about the disc result from occlusion of major choroidal arteries.[473] Similar pigment blotches have been produced experimentally in the cat by injection of emboli into the posterior ciliary arteries.[307]

Flat mounts of the choroidal vessels cannot be prepared by trypsin digestion as well as for the retinal vessels because of the collagen-rich extraneous tissue.

Unlike the retinal arteries, those in the choroid show typical atheromatosis. This is, in fact, the commonest cause of occlusion of the larger choroidal vessels. On the other hand, the common cause for occlusion of the smaller arteries is hypertension. Other documented causes of choroidal artery occlusion are polyarteritis and cardiac myxomata (p. 124).

SECONDARY

Carotid Artery Stenosis

Stenosis and occlusion of the carotid artery are a common cause of cerebrovascular accidents (25 per cent according to one series)[199] and have significant ophthalmic manifestions.[123, 293, 326, 341, 370, 395, 569] Ocular symptoms are present in some 65 per cent of patients with carotid insufficiency.[325] The usual site of obstruction is the bifurcation of the common carotid[261] at the level of the C4 and C5 vertebrae but may be anywhere along the carotid system (Fig. 95). Atheromatosis is the

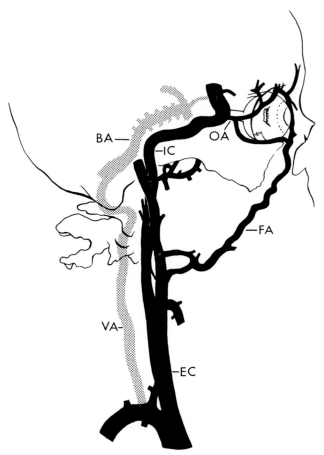

Figure 95   Carotid circulation illustrating alternate route of blood supply to the brain. In the event of an obstruction in the internal carotid artery, blood may reach the brain by way of the external carotid artery (instead of the internal carotid), the facial artery, and the ophthalmic artery through the orbit. *EC*, external carotid; *FA*, facial artery; *OA*, ophthalmic artery; *IC*, internal carotid; *VA*, vertebral artery; *BA*, basilar artery.

usual cause in middle-aged or older persons but trauma, inflammation, or congenital defects may be responsible at a younger age.[350] Carotid obstruction is said to be more than twice as common in males as in females and affects the left side six to seven times as frequently as the right side.[207]

The symptoms of carotid occlusion are hemiplegia (or other signs of cerebral ischemia) on the contralateral side of the body, recurrent visual blur leading at times to monocular blindness on the homolateral side,[206, 265] decreased carotid pulsation, a bruit, and a slow rate of filling of the vessels by fluoroangiography. When present, a lower retinal blood pressure on the ipsilateral side is corroborative evidence[39, 341, 698] but is not always present (see ophthalmodynamometry, p. 27). Arteriography provides the definitive diagnosis and indicates the site of the lesion.[149, 406]

When retinal diastolic measurements fail to reveal a carotid occlusion, determination of the systolic pressure,[478, 609] as well as comparative measurements with the patient in the supine and erect positions,[325, 607] may be informative. A carotid compression test[673] has been recommended in which the retinal pressures are measured with and without compression of the intact carotid. In patients who have developed crossed collateral circulation, such a maneuver will result in fall of the retinal pressures in *both* eyes. This test is, however, somewhat dangerous, as it occludes the entire carotid circulation; it is not, therefore, generally used (p. 27).

Occasionally the fundus will show cotton-wool spots and typical occlusion of the central retinal artery[144, 612] or an ischemic optic neuropathy.[73] The incidence of central artery occlusion has been variously estimated as from 4 to 16 per cent.[325, 479] With simple lowering of the central artery pressure, the fundus picture may be that of a venous stasis retinopathy.[370]

While the ocular signs with carotid occlusion are those of ischemia, they may be due to occult emboli from carotid plaques ("rough plaques" by arteriography)[261] and not, as was at one time believed, necessarily due to the lower blood pressure. The emboli are often cryptogenic and on occasion may be seen traversing the retinal vascular system.[204]

If the retinal artery shows a significantly lower pressure in one eye but still has a crisp pulsation, the obstruction is presumably in the carotid system. On the other hand, equal pressures in the two sides with a poor pulsation and delayed refilling on one side indicates a local obstruction in the ophthalmic system.[607, 609]

Although approximately half of the patients with carotid occlusion have visual disturbances, only 10 per cent develop blindness in the eye.[359] The presence or absence of ophthalmic signs depends largely on the rate with which the obstruction has occurred and the site of obstruction. When the carotid occlusion has developed slowly, collateral circulation may bypass the obstruction effectively, giving no ophthalmic indication of the stenosis and yielding deceptively equal retinal artery pressures.[611] This collateral circulation may be by way of the external carotid artery[344, 439, 455] with rich anastomoses in the orbit[246] when the obstruction is in the internal carotid artery, or it may be by way of the opposite internal carotid artery, with retrograde flow in the ipsilateral carotid, when the obstruction involves the common carotid. The more peripheral the obstruction the less effective is the collateral circulation.

With obstruction of the middle cerebral artery or obstruction of the internal carotid distal to its ophthalmic branch, the retinal artery pressures may be actually higher on the involved side.

When both common carotid arteries are occluded, collateral circulation may derive from the posterior cerebral system, provided that the stenosis has occurred sufficiently slowly and that the patient has been sufficiently youthful to have had plastic vessels.

Suggestive of an uncompensated or incompletely compensated carotid occlusion are the intermittent visual symptoms associated with fluctuation in the blood pressure.[144] Thus blackouts in one eye and crossed hemiplegia, often designated as transient ischemic attacks, may be the presenting signs of a carotid stenosis and antedate the final occlusion by months or years. These attacks may be precipitated by emotional stress or other vascular crises. They go on to permanent blindness in 15 to 25 per cent of cases.[207, 359] Curiously, the blackouts which occur with stenosis of the internal carotid artery cease when the vessel becomes completely occluded.[325]

Recognizing carotid stenosis early is important because it can be effectively treated. An estimated 80 per cent develop hemiplegia if untreated.[207] Anticoagulants will abort the transient attacks,[476] while endarterectomy and bypass surgery will provide a cure in suitable cases.

A special case of occlusion of the carotids (and of other arteries) in women is that occurring with fibromuscular dysplasia.[294] In this case both carotids may be severely stenotic with characteristic "beading" in the arteriograms,[338, 339] but since it comes on at an early age and develops slowly, the ischemic symptoms are remarkably slight.

Aortic Arch Syndrome

The aortic arch syndrome, one of the pulseless diseases, is a hypotensive condition resulting from stenosis of the major branches of the aorta. The arteries involved are particularly the innominate, the subclavian, the carotid, and the vertebral branches.[638] The symptoms are those of a functional ischemia of the areas supplied by the most stenosed arteries. Their diversity can be best appreciated by refer-

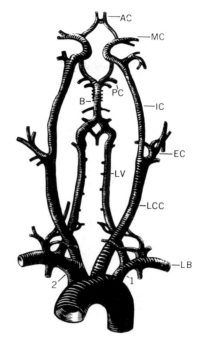

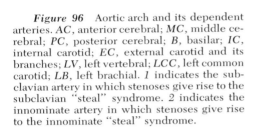

Figure 96 Aortic arch and its dependent arteries. *AC*, anterior cerebral; *MC*, middle cerebral; *PC*, posterior cerebral; *B*, basilar; *IC*, internal carotid; *EC*, external carotid and its branches; *LV*, left vertebral; *LCC*, left common carotid; *LB*, left brachial. *1* indicates the subclavian artery in which stenoses give rise to the subclavian "steal" syndrome. *2* indicates the innominate artery in which stenoses give rise to the innominate "steal" syndrome.

ence to the accompanying diagram (Fig. 96). Prominent are the weak or absent pulses in the arms and neck and the relationship of the patients' symptoms to posture. At times the patients may be unable to sit or stand without fainting. The pathogenesis of these symptoms is similar to that of simple carotid occlusion but differs in the site affected and thereby in the multiplicity of arteries involved. The common cause is atheromatosis but an arteritis (see Takayasu's disease, p. 134) or any obliterative disease of the aortic arch (syphilis, trauma) may be the cause.[553]

The ophthalmic symptoms of the aortic arch syndrome are often prominent.[641] Increasingly frequent blackouts related to posture are common. The fundi are apt to show spontaneous arterial pulsation (with low ophthalmic dynamometric measurements), narrowing of the arteries, distension of the veins, slow circulation (evident by fluoroangiography or boxcar segmentation of blood), cotton-wool spots, hemorrhages, and a characteristic plethora of microaneurysms.[166] Cataracts, appearing two to four years after the onset of ischemic symptoms, seem to be characteristic[303] and to be due to associated involvement of the ciliary circulation. Occasionally the entire eye will be involved, with iris necrosis in addition to the retinal ischemia.[450]

The microaneurysms differ from those of diabetes in being uniformly small and situated at the bifurcation of the capillaries rather than saccular outpouchings along the walls of the capillaries. They have been well demon-strated histopathologically.[188, 473]

The evolution of the aortic arch syndrome is usually gradual; hence it reaches a pulseless state while still compatible with life. However, a rapidly developing and usually fatal syndrome occurs when a dissecting aortic aneurysm blocks the major vessels.[87]

Variants of the aortic arch syndrome induce combinations of arm and leg symptoms. Especially noteworthy are the syndromes that occur with occlusion of either the subclavian artery on the left[546] or the innominate artery on the right.[632] In such cases the blood supply may be shunted as a reverse flow down the corresponding vertebral artery to the ipsilateral arm. Because blood is thus stolen from the posterior cerebral circulation, the syndromes are called the subclavian steal and the innominate steal syndromes. The symptoms arise from ischemia of the posterior cerebral area; hence they are discussed with lesions of the occipital lobes (see p. 152). Most characteristic of these steal syndromes is transient hemianopia or blindness, sometimes precipi-tated by use of the arm[493] and accompanied by vertigo, paresthesias, and limb paralysis.[198] Corroborative of this diagnosis is a significant in-equality in the blood pressure of the two arms, but proof depends on the radiographic demonstration of reverse flow in the vertebral-caro-tid systems.

A further variant of the aortic arch syndrome is the arteritis occur-ring most frequently in oriental young women (see Takayasu's dis-ease, p. 134). Its symptoms are similar to those of atheromatous origin and are also included with pulseless disease.

Sickle Cell Disease, Thalassemia, and Eales' Disease

SICKLE CELL DISEASE. Retinopathy is frequent with sickle cell abnormalities. The small (5 μ) and relatively rigid capillaries of the retina make it a target organ for obstruction by the altered red blood cells. The deoxygenated sickle cells can no longer mold into the paraboloid shapes that are necessary for transit through the capillaries and obstruction occurs in the microcirculatory bed.

The minimal manifestations of sickle cell retinopathy are tor-tuosity of the retinal veins, arteriolar occlusions, and arteriovenous anastomoses.[118, 253, 677] These produce no symptoms. Hemorrhages into the retina and occasionally into the vitreous herald more severe ob-structive disease.[172, 286, 311, 604] Retinal or vitreous hemorrhages are often the presenting symptoms. Fluoroangiography will usually show a diffuse leakage of dye. The terminal retinal arterioles and venules become ensheathed (sometimes chalk-white),[262, 263] as occurs with any obstructive vascular disease in the retina. These changes are apt to be

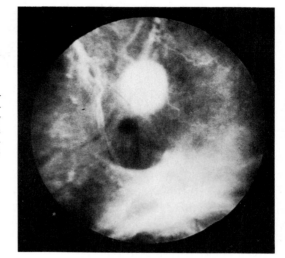

Figure 97 Proliferative retinopathy with sickle cell hemoglobinopathy. The feathery opacities represent scar tissue in the vitreous while the white circle represents the blurred image of the optic disc.

most evident in the temporal periphery, possibly owing to their remoteness in the retinal circulation. The entire central retinal artery may be occluded.[472] Finally, retinal proliferation occurs, similar to that in diabetes, with detachment of the retina[253, 262, 529] and frequently secondary glaucoma (Fig. 97). Less obvious are changes in the choroidal arteries (which may occur in infancy)[622] that ultimately result in the black sunburst sign of choroidal infarction (see p. 64).

Angioid streaks, which, as described elsewhere (see p. 96), are due to ruptures of Bruch's membrane, may occur with sickle cell disease of either the SS or SC variety.[243, 505] The basis for this association is unknown.

The ocular pathology in sickle cell disease is similar to that of other forms of hemorrhagic retinopathy. It is characterized by occlusive vascular changes and detachment of the retina.[63, 243, 262] Lipid and cholesterol deposits, similar to what one finds in diabetes and Coats' disease, have also been surprisingly conspicuous.

Whether all sickle cell hemoglobinopathies produce the same retinal changes, varying only in degree, or whether different hemoglobinopathies evoke different types of retinopathy is an important but unsettled question. Some observers have equated the ocular manifestations of SS and SC disease,[430] while others, in an extensive study, have correlated the electrophoretic patterns with different types of retinopathy. Specifically, the vascular proliferations into the vitreous ("sea fans") from the peripheral retina are thought to be characteristic of SC hemoglobinopathy while focal degenerations producing pigmented areas (black sunbursts) are thought to be characteristic of SS hemoglobinopathy.[252, 677] These pigmented spots probably indicate involvement of the choroidal vasculature.

Curiously, the retinal changes with the more severe SS disease produce less serious visual disturbances than do the hemorrhagic and proliferative disturbances of the milder SC disease. Moreover, retinal detachment, secondary glaucoma, and necrosis of the eye following surgery appear to be more common with SC than with SS retinopathy.[564]

The hemorrhagic and proliferative types of sickle cell retinopathy are progressive. Medical therapy (anticoagulation) has not been beneficial. Photocoagulation is, therefore, the treatment of choice if the bleeding points or new formed vessels can be identified and are accessible to the coagulative beam. The argon laser is presently the instrument of choice. This not only occludes the vessels but also welds the retina to the choroid so as to prevent detachment.

THALASSEMIA. Thalassemic hemoglobinopathy may produce the same type of retinopathy as does sickle cell (SC) hemoglobinopathy.[256] This consists of vascular occlusions, retinal and vitreous hemorrhages,[640] and detachment of the retina.[364, 558] Since the minor form is compatible with otherwise normal activity, the retinopathy may be a presenting symptom. The pathogenesis of the ocular vasculopathy is obscure since thalassemia is not known to produce intravascular obstruction as does sickle cell disease.

EALES' DISEASE. Eales' disease[171] is a vaso-obliterative disease of the retina which has a superficial resemblance to sickle cell and thalassemic retinopathy but has no other association with these entities nor proved linkage to systemic disease.[169] It occurs predominantly in young adult males and may present with a vitreous hemorrhage. As the vitreous clears, the retinal periphery reveals hemorrhages within the retina and white threads replacing the arteries and veins. It may eventually be bilateral and can, through organization of the retina, lead to vitreous fibrosis, retinal detachment, and blindness. More frequently, however, it remains an occlusive vasculopathy in the retinal periphery and may be asymptomatic.[163]

The cause of Eales' disease is unknown but a vast literature has at different times attributed it to tuberculosis, Buerger's obliterative angiitis, and focal infection. It has been reported in association with intracranial and spinal cord lesions.[46, 594, 650] No hemoglobinopathy has been demonstrated despite the resemblance to sickle cell disease. It is commonly included with inflammatory diseases and termed *periphlebitis retinae* but evidence for this etiology is generally lacking.

Treatment of Eales' disease with steroids has been recommended[174, 175] but the results are difficult to evaluate. Surface diathermy[163] or photocoagulation[176] is indicated for the associated proliferative vasculopathy.

Retrolental Fibroplasia

Despite its name, the entity called retrolental fibroplasia is initially neither retrolental nor fibroplastic. It is a retinal vasculopathy of premature infants induced by excessive ambient oxygen during incubation.[82, 191, 377, 511, 539] It is an incubator disease affecting infants less than four pounds birth weight and has been, in the last quarter century, a prolific cause of blindness.

The first clinical evidences of the disease are dilatation of the peripheral vessels,[485] hemorrhages into the peripheral retina and vitreous, and neovasculogenesis from the peripheral retina.[512] These occur within a few weeks after the baby is removed from the incubator.[501, 646] The condition may then be arrested spontaneously or, alternatively, the retina may be pulled toward one side, grossly distorting the vessels, to produce the appearance known as "dragged discs" (Fig. 98).[47] Vision is then considerably impaired. In the more severe cases, the recurrent hemorrhages and neovasculogenesis into the vitreous lead to a detachment of the retina with corresponding gliosis and to the final retrolental mass that gave this condition the name of retrolental fibroplasia.[636] Progressive traction on the retina and detachment, or retinoschisis (splitting of the retina),[92] may continue for years after birth.[192]

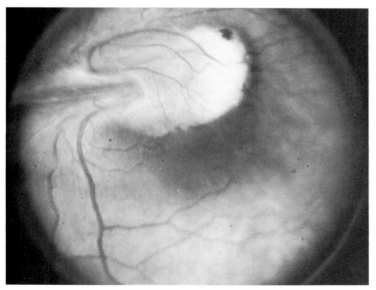

Figure 98   "Dragged disc" in retrolental fibroplasia. Tissue containing the retinal blood vessels extends from the disc to the nasal periphery.

The patient was a 23 year old girl who as a premature baby had had prolonged incubation in a high oxygen atmosphere. Her vision in the eye illustrated here was reduced to counting fingers whereas she was totally blind in the other eye from detachment of the retina.

The pathogenesis of retrolental fibroplasia has been well documented and found to depend on the growth pattern of retinal vessels in the newborn. By the time of birth, the retinal vessels of the premature infant have not yet extended to the periphery.[97] Oxygen causes, temporarily, a contraction of the arteries and cessation in growth of the vessels but the retina itself continues to grow. When, after days or weeks in the incubator, the infant is returned to normal atmospheric oxygen, the arteries reopen but apparently cannot resume their extension into the peripheral retina. Instead, they penetrate the then thin internal limiting membrane and proliferate into the vitreous.[33] Such neovasculogenic vessels have extremely thin walls and are prone to leak with the march of symptoms described above. The severity of the condition is, in general, proportional to the state of prematurity.[15]

An analogous retinopathy has been produced in animals with excessive oxygen[276] and found to depend on spasm of the retinal arteries.[33, 510] Significantly, it occurs in immature but not mature animals.

No other vessel in the body appears to share the devastating effects of oxygen excess as does the retinal system. Even the choroid fails to show a comparable vasculopathy.[511] However, the infants often do have other abnormalities associated with prematurity.

The treatment of retrolental fibroplasia is largely prophylactic. Infants should be exposed to excessive oxygen only as long as it is necessary for maintenance of life. Precautions now in operation have greatly reduced, although not eliminated, the incidence of retrolental fibroplasia.[91, 705]

Miscellaneous Occlusive Arterial Disease

Incorporated under this heading are several unrelated entities some of which, although unquestionably occlusive, are too infrequent to warrant more than passing mention and others of which are only questionably occlusive in nature.

What might be called the "retinal steal syndrome" occurs occasionally when blood is robbed from the retina to supply an orbital or para-orbital tumor[699] or when, in the presence of an occluded carotid artery, collateral flow through the external carotid passes in a reverse direction through the ophthalmic artery to the cerebral circulation.[571] In either case blackouts occur at the time of retinal ischemia and sometimes result in permanent blindness.

Homocystinuria, which is known to cause occlusion of the medium-sized arteries of the body, has been reported to cause occlusion of the retinal arteries in association with glaucoma.[685]

The collagenoses that have been reported to cause retinal artery occlusion include polyarteritis[190, 685] and disseminated lupus erythematosus. The hyperviscosity syndromes and cryoglobulinemia[181] may be associated with arterial occlusion although venous occlusion is more likely (see p. 130).

Central serous retinopathy must be mentioned, if for no other reason than that it is frequently called "angiospastic retinopathy" and is sometimes confused with optic neuritis and other causes of central scotomas. It consists of serous exudate from the choriocapillaris that raises the pigment epithelium and retina. Ophthalmoscopy shows only subtle elevation of the retina but fluoroangiography reveals the exudate well and often discloses a pinpoint leak (see Fig. 21, p. 26).

Since central serous retinopathy involves preferentially the central portion of the fundus, vision is impaired but the visual loss is usually reversible. The condition is frequently recurrent, however, and progressive forms merging into disciform degeneration are not infrequent. It occurs predominately in young males, especially those of a compulsive temperament; hence it has been likened to angioneurotic edema, but there is no evidence to support an angiopathic etiology.

A rarer but possibly related entity is multifocal placoid epitheliopathy.[236] This is a bilateral, benign condition which is ordinarily of ophthalmic significance only but has been reported once in association with erythema nodosum.[647]

The crinkled retina syndrome (or pre-retinal macular fibrosis)[689] is characterized by distorted and impaired vision of minor degree with irregularities of the ophthalmoscopic highlights from the central retina.[381] The macular vessels become abnormally tortuous. The condition involves one or both eyes of middle-aged or older persons but is not necessarily progressive. Histologically it consists of folds of the internal limiting membrane and a thin overlying cellular layer.[351, 457, 473, 630] The pathogenesis is obscure. The reasons for including it in the present category are the suggestion of an underlying occlusive vascular disease[689] and an alleged significant association with diabetes.[554]

Microcystic macular dystrophy is initially an edema of the macula resulting from leakage out of the perifoveal capillaries. It is especially common in eyes which have had a cataract extraction and often occurs at the time of rupture of the anterior vitreous face.[349] It is then known as the Irvine-Gass syndrome.[239, 349] The diagnosis can best be made by fluoroangiography which reveals the perimacular leak and a characteristic star-shaped staining of the macula.[238] The condition is usually reversible but it may, on the other hand, lead to a permanent cystoid degeneration of the macula. Its pathogenesis is unknown. The unilaterality and relationship to surgery suggest a strictly local process, but an association with cardiovascular disease and hypertension has been claimed.[239]

A perennial question is whether or not any form of macular degeneration can be ascribed to disturbances of the retinal circulation. In the lay mind "hardening of the arteries" provides an easy explanation. Some surveys suggest a high incidence of senile macular dystrophy with venous occlusion,[537] and obliterative changes in the perifoveal capillaries have been found late (but not early) in senile macular degenerations.[403] Yet macular degeneration is not a regular feature of occlusive vascular disease, and it seems unlikely that macular degeneration results from occlusive vascular disease in the retina.

EMBOLIC

Emboli, or more precisely microemboli, are a frequent cause of retinal artery occlusions. The symptoms they produce, their ophthalmoscopic appearance, and to some extent their prognostic implications vary with the nature of the embolic material.

Calcific

The common sources of calcific emboli are vegetations from rheumatic valvular disease of the heart[179, 520] and atheromatous plaques in the carotid artery or aorta. They are especially apt to follow the manipulations of surgical valvulotomy[331] but may occur without apparent provocation.

The one ophthalmic symptom is blindness. This may involve the entire eye or a field corresponding to the obstructed artery. It is often accompanied by hemiplegia or hemisensory symptoms of the contralateral half of the body due to simultaneous embolization to the brain. The fundus shows the typical opacification of the retina, cherry red spot, and narrowing of arteries as occur with any retinal artery occlusion.

Emboli may or may not be seen in the fundus. The usual site where the emboli become lodged is just posterior to the lamina cribrosa and here they are invisible by ophthalmoscopy. The examiner then has no way, short of studying the enucleated eye, to know that the occlusion was embolic in origin. However, the embolus may move on to the nerve head (Fig. 99) or fragments of it may split off to pass into the retinal vessels. Calcific emboli rarely move far from the disc.

In surprising contrast to the critical onset and relatively stationary course of these calcific emboli is the account of frequent obscurations of vision in patients with rheumatic heart disease who are presumed to have recurrent showers of emboli.[624]

The calcific emboli are characteristically mat white, non-scintillating, and somewhat wider than the blood column. Those on the

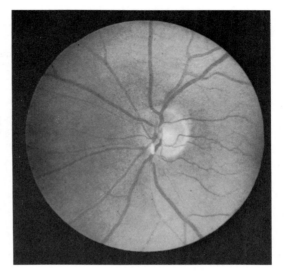

Figure 99 Embolus lodged in the inferior temporal artery on the nerve head.

disc are often overlooked because they merge into the white background but those in the retina stand out conspicuously against the orange flush.

The retinal arteries may convert into white threads when the impacted emboli cause permanent occlusion of the artery but often the circulation is restored surprisingly rapidly as the embolus is either exteriorized or bypassed by collateral circulation. Although this does not ordinarily occur rapidly enough to have any beneficial effect on vision, it does restore the circulation to what appears to be normal.

Surprisingly few pathologic studies of calcific emboli have been reported. These few have shown the preferred position of the embolus at the lamina cribrosa or in the peripapillary region (Fig. 100). The artery has been occluded and the retina infarcted. Occasionally emboli have also been found in the posterior ciliary arteries.[41] One case which began with the unusual feature of a vitreous hemorrhage was found to have an embolus that encroached on the adjacent vein.[103]

Lipid

Emboli of lipid material usually originate in an atheroma of a stenotic carotid artery.[325, 326] They may occur spontaneously, presumably from an internal ulceration of the artery, or may result from either trauma to the neck or manipulation of the artery at the time of arteriography[109, 271, 285, 484] or endarterectomy.[326, 587] One case resulted merely from the manipulation of stethoscopy.[654]

While causing a similar infarction of the retina, lipid emboli differ from calcific emboli in that they are yellowish, scintillating, and mul-

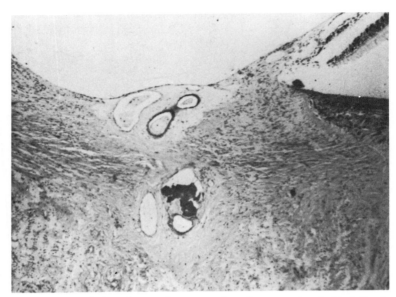

Figure 100 Embolus of central artery within the nerve just behind the lamina cribrosa. (Hematoxylin-eosin stain.)

tiple, and lodge at the bifurcations of the retinal arteries (especially of the superior temporal branch; Fig. 101).[477] They are also more apt to be transient. At times they can be followed in their movement downstream to a more peripheral branch or into the capillary bed. Often they pass through the vascular system entirely, leaving only zones of retinal opacity or reversible changes in their wake.[274, 409] At other times cholesterol emboli may lodge at an arterial bifurcation without

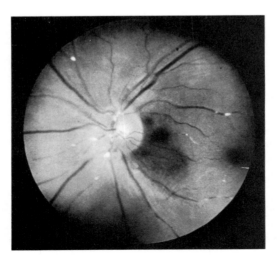

Figure 101 Multiple lipid emboli.

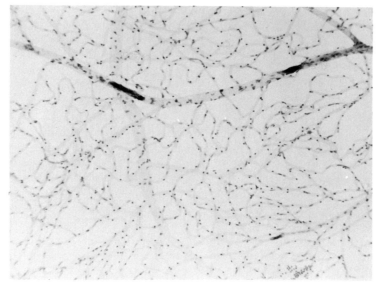

Figure 102 Lipid emboli in arteriole. (Flat mount prepared by trypsin digestion and stained with Sudan-hematoxylin.)

obstructing the lumen and, therefore, without causing any symptoms.[326]

Some cases of amaurosis fugax are undoubtedly caused by showers of lipid emboli. These showers have actually been witnessed on several occasions.[328] What were at one time interpreted as atheromatous plaques may actually be emboli.[204, 322, 329, 706]

A special instance of lipid emboli occurs with crushing injury to the long bones and chest. This, known as Purtscher's disease, is manifest in the fundi by cotton-wool spots, retinal edema, and hemorrhages.[229, 368] The emboli are inconspicuous clinically but have been demonstrated pathologically.[148, 368]

Histopathologic demonstration of lipid emboli has been reported in a few cases (Fig. 102). The malleable emboli adjust themselves to the lumen of the vessels with surprisingly little trauma to the adjacent wall and little phagocytosis. They consist of neutral fat and cholesterol.[109, 135]

Platelet-Fibrinous

Some of the circulating emboli which are seen to pass through the vessels[204, 333, 560, 709] with either blindness or transient visual obscurations are believed to be composed of platelets.[20, 560, 561, 601] They occur significantly with thrombocytosis and may be abolished by aspirin.[484] A similar fundus appearance has been produced by injection of platelets or ADP into the circulation.[504]

The emboli which follow myocardial infarction, and possibly those associated with mucor thrombi as well,[103] probably fall into the category of fibrin plugs.[706] They are especially frequent in persons who develop neurologic complications with open heart surgery.[684]

Myxomatous

An occasional source for emboli is the myxomata of the heart. These tumors have a preference for the left atrium and are often unsuspected until they produce peripheral symptoms through tumor emboli. Several cases of embolic occlusion of the central retinal artery have been reported clinically[487, 543, 596] and two cases have been studied pathologically.[103, 448] Such an etiology should be suspected when occlusion of the central artery occurs in a young person without evidence of rheumatic heart disease, marantic endocarditis, or other source for the emboli. The symptoms from these myxomatous emboli are commonly mistaken for those of subacute bacterial endocarditis.[627]

Since cardiac myxomata are now accessible to surgery,[708] once the diagnosis is made, and since they are otherwise fatal, the possibility of myxomatous emboli must be kept in mind.[452]

The diagnosis may be suggested by cardiac auscultation (although easily confused with mitral stenosis) and confirmed either by cardiac arteriography or by biopsy of an affected artery. It may also be suggested by finding multiple and diffuse aneurysms in cerebral angiograms.[488]

The histopathology of the emboli is like that of the original tumor and pathognomonic of the source. It consists of stellate cells in an abundantly mucoid matrix with or without invasion of the arterial wall. The slow growing and benign nature of these tumors does not permit a conclusion as to whether they act simply as plugs or actually proliferate in situ.

Experimental

Experimental embolization has been studied in the retina of the cat[30] and pig[35, 161, 583] using latex[241] and glass spheres. This has permitted the sequential study of flow patterns and of the development of collateral circulation about microinfarcts. Fluoroangiography has shown that the first evidence of collateral circulation occurs in 35 minutes but is not well developed until four days and not complete for several weeks. Large vascular channels developing from preexisting capillaries acquire a cellularity similar to that of normal arterioles and ultimately restore the circulation to the previously infarcted area.

Retinal emboli have been produced in the monkey by injection of air[549] or fibrin[409, 504] with resultant fluorescein leakage attributed to endothelial damage. Cholesterol injection has resulted in scintillating emboli similar to those occurring in human beings.[329]

SUMMARY

Occlusion of the central retinal artery causes a sudden blindness which may be permanent even though some circulation is shortly re-established. When the patient is first examined, a loss of the crisp retinal pulse and boxcar segmentation of the blood column may be the only abnormalities, but after a few hours cloudy swelling of the ganglion cells will result in the classic cherry red spot. Of the many causes of retinal artery occlusion, atheromatosis of the central artery in the optic nerve and embolus are the most common. The site of involvement is usually the lamina cribrosa.

Ischemic optic neuropathy, on the other hand, is due to occlusion of the posterior ciliary arteries resulting most commonly from atheromatosis (presumably) or temporal arteritis. The typical fundus picture is papilledema with or without pallor of the disc and a few papillary hemorrhages. Its appearance can scarcely be differentiated from papillitis.

Because of their relative inaccessibility, occlusions of the choroidal arteries have been less well documented. The ophthalmoscope usually reveals simply pigmentary disturbances.

Secondary retinal artery occlusion is frequently caused by carotid stenosis and is sometimes associated with contralateral hemiplegia. The occlusion may result from the hypotension but is often associated with emboli. When the stenosis develops gradually, collateral circulation through either the external carotid or the circle of Willis may effectively prevent visual symptoms from developing. The aortic arch syndrome may produce similar ischemic attacks in the retina but the episodes are more obviously related to hypotension and associated with abnormal pulses in the arms. Various steal syndromes result in occipital ischemia with resultant transient hemianopia or blindness.

The small size and thick walls of the retinal capillaries predispose them to obstruction by sickled cells with resultant hemorrhages, vascular proliferation, and detachment of the retina. Thalassemia and the ocular condition known as Eales' disease may induce similar retinal pictures although the pathogenesis in both cases is obscure.

Retrolental fibroplasia is the result of aberrant neovascularization in the eyes of premature babies sub ected to high oxygen tension. It has been a common cause of blindness but is not regularly associated with other defects.

Other occlusive arterial diseases of the retina include: steal syndromes in which blood is robbed from the retina to supply orbital masses, homocystinuria in which the retinal artery participates with other arterial disease, and the collagenoses and hyperviscosity syndromes. There are also several entities which are questionably relevant to arterial occlusion. These include central serous retinopathy, a crinkled retina syndrome, microcystic macular dystrophy, and other forms of macular degeneration.

The two most common types of emboli obstructing retinal arteries are calcific emboli coming from either rheumatic vegetations on the heart valves or calcific plaques in the carotid artery and lipid emboli coming from atheromatous ulcerations in the carotid or cardiac walls.

Calcific emboli usually lodge at the lamina cribrosa and are not ophthalmoscopically visible but fragments may enter the retinal arteries to lodge near the disc. Usually no more than one or two are visible and these have a characteristically mat white color. Lipid emboli, on the other hand, are typically multiple, yellowish, and often scintillating. They lodge particularly at the arterial bifurcation and may or may not be obstructive.

Emboli made up of fibrin and platelets contribute to the circulating emboli that cause transient blackouts but may result in permanent blindness. They occur with thrombocytosis, myocardial infarction, and bypass surgery on the heart.

Cardiac myxomata comprise a rare but important source of retinal emboli whose clinical recognition may be lifesaving.

CHAPTER 7

OCCLUSIVE VENOUS DISEASE OF THE EYE

PRIMARY

Occlusion of the retinal veins comprises the most common vascular accident in the eye. Its cause is not usually apparent on clinical examination and hence is designated primary, but what is clinically primary may have several histopathologic explanations.

Venous occlusion usually induces rapid loss of vision, sometimes first observed on awaking in the morning, but it may be preceded by episodes of blurred vision[384] and photopsia. Unlike central artery occlusion, however, the visual loss is not total. Light perception and sometimes perception of hand movements are maintained. One should suspect coexistent occlusion of the artery when vision is lost entirely.[537] At times the patient volunteers that the background has a reddish discoloration.

The ophthalmoscopic picture in total occlusion is striking. The entire fundus is replaced by hemorrhages through which the dark, distended, and tortuous veins alternately emerge and disappear (Fig. 103). The disc is swollen and all but hidden by the hemorrhages which obliterate its margins and extend to its center. Cotton-wool spots are present but usually inconspicuous. If the hemorrhages have extended into the vitreous, the entire fundus may be hidden from view.

The hemorrhages gradually absorb and the retinal veins return to more nearly normal dimensions, but very slowly. The resolving process may, in fact, require two to three years. The veins then show an ensheathing of their walls and a corkscrew tortuosity of the small vessels. This latter represents collateral vessels and is especially conspicuous about the disc, forming a corona, or caput medusae, that connects the retinal and choroidal circulation.

An especially dreaded complication, occurring in approximately

127

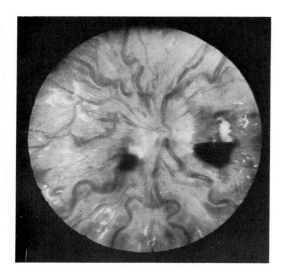

Figure 103 Occlusion of the central retinal vein.

one quarter of all cases of central vein occlusion (and occasionally of artery occlusion[522]) is the development of new formed vessels on the iris (rubeosis iridis) and in the angle of the anterior chamber. This results in glaucoma[537] after several months (the "100 day glaucoma" of Coats[95]). This hemorrhagic glaucoma is not amenable to treatment and most eyes with this condition have to be removed eventually on account of pain.

The site of obstruction with central vein occlusion is at the lamina cribrosa. The vein is here compressed by the fibrous membrane and by the adjacent artery with which it often shares a common adventitia. The immediate cause of the obstruction has been generally assumed to be either thrombosis[94] or endothelial proliferation.[651] Histopathologic evidence has been presented supporting both possibilities.[187, 382, 389, 579] In either case the pressure from sclerotic arterial changes predisposes the vein to occlusion.[578]

Branch or tributary venous occlusion occurs characteristically at an arteriovenous crossing and causes initially a fan-shaped distribution of hemorrhages that radiate out from this crossing (Fig. 104). The superior temporal branch is the one most commonly affected. The degree of visual loss depends on how much of the macula is involved by the associated cystoid edema or hole formation in the retina.[65] Venous occlusions toward the periphery may be asymptomatic or cause only a shower of floaters when the hemorrhages extend into the vitreous.

The late manifestations of branch occlusion are ensheathing of the affected vein, sometimes with replacement by a white line; microaneurysms in the distribution of the obstructed vein; and various collaterals circumventing the arteriovenous point of obstruc-

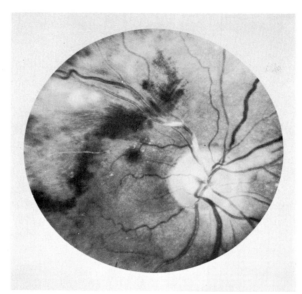

Figure 104 Tributary venous occlusion. The site of obstruction is an AV crossing of the superior temporal vessels and is associated with local opacification of the arterial wall.

tion (Fig. 105). All these manifestations stand out conspicuously in fluoroangiograms. The microaneurysms become increasingly prominent with a pattern like lights on a Christmas tree.

The rubeosis iridis and glaucoma which occur so frequently with central vein occlusion rarely occur with branch occlusions.

Eales' disease, which has been previously discussed with arterial occlu-

Figure 105 Pattern of collateral venules that bypass a tributary venous obstruction. The arrow indicates an occluded vessel.

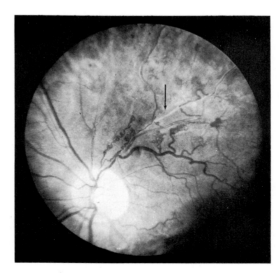

sions (see p. 116), often begins with venous occlusion and was originally described as a cause of vitreous hemorrhage.

Numerous histopathologic studies of advanced cases of central vein occlusion have revealed the obstruction at the lamina cribrosa. Depending on the duration of the occlusion the retinas have shown either massive hemorrhages or severe gliosis and hemosiderosis. Flat mounts of the retinal vessels show nonspecific occlusion (acellularity) of many capillaries, venovenular shunts, and a floral-like display of microaneurysms on the venular side of the capillary bed.[417]

Treatment of venous obstruction has its enthusiastic[389, 649, 689] and skeptical[676] advocates for anticoagulant and thrombolytic agents.[431, 436] Prophylactic anticoagulation for threatened venous occlusion has the theoretical merit of forestalling any acute episode and thereby providing time for the development of collateral circulation. Low molecular dextrons have also been recommended.[534] Recurrent bleeding points, however, are best treated by photocoagulation.

SECONDARY

Secondary venous occlusion and stasis differ from the primary type only insofar as a cause is clinically recognizable. Diabetes is a prime predisposing cause.[13, 76] Other specific entities are polycythemia,[56, 65, 555, 575] hyperglobulinemia,[134] cryoglobulinemia,[12, 193] multiple myeloma,[189, 440] Raynaud's disease,[686] and macroglobulinemia,[1, 14, 31, 575, 616] in all of which an underlying hyperviscosity may be the significant factor (Fig. 106).[54, 84, 210] Isolated instances of venous occlusion have also been reported with a tubercle (presumed tuberculosis)[566, 653] and Boeck's sarcoid.[429] Whether or not estrogens ("the pill") may cause occlusion of the retinal vein (or artery) is a current controversy that has not been settled but some reports suggest that it may at least cause retinal edema.[263, 668] Venous occlusion with vasculitis, sickle cell disease, Eales' disease, and thalassemia are discussed elsewhere (see p. 114), since they are also associated with arterial obstructions.

The precipitating cause for the occlusion is often a slowing of the circulation from either an occlusion of the retinal artery or a drop in blood pressure causing a stagnation thrombosis.[300, 382] Thus, some 5 per cent of patients with carotid artery stenosis have a venous stasis retinopathy.[302, 370, 641] For the same reason it may be a feature of hypertension or arteriosclerosis which causes retinal artery stenosis.

Yet the most common cause of venous occlusion in eyes that come to the pathology laboratory is not vascular disease at all but glaucoma. The elevated intraocular pressure impairs the outflow of blood by occluding the vein at its exit and thereby causing stasis.[537]

Partial venous obstruction is more frequent with the hyperviscosity syndromes than is total occlusion. The retinal picture then con-

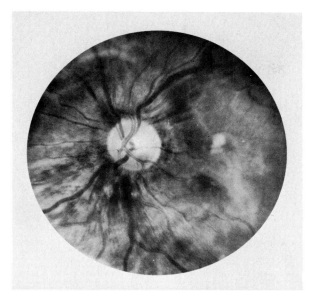

Figure 106   Venous obstruction with macroglobulinemia (hyperviscosity retino-pathy).

sists of dilatation of the veins, papilledema, occasional boxcar segmentation of the blood column induced by gentle pressure on the eye,[360] a scattering of hemorrhages, microaneurysms,[26, 31] and cotton-wool spots.[7, 122, 332, 575] These are present in both eyes and are approximately symmetric. The associated systemic symptoms include bleeding from mucous membranes, cyanosis, vertigo, deafness, cardiac failure, and various neurologic symptoms (the last of which is called the Bing-Neal syndrome).

SUMMARY

Acute occlusion of the retinal vein, the most common vascular accident in the eye, presents an unmistakable fundus picture of greatly distended veins and massive retinal hemorrhages. Chronic occlusion results in various patterns of collateral channels that bypass the obstruction which is usually situated at an arteriovenous crossing. Treatment is largely ineffectual. A frequent late complication of central vein occlusion is a severe form of glaucoma that requires enucleation on account of pain.

The underlying causes of venous occlusion are multiple. Diabetes ranks high on the list, and the various hyperviscosity syndromes are also frequent causes. A local vasculitis may present with venous occlusion. In addition, slowing of the circulation through arterial disease or through elevation of the intraocular pressure may be the precipitating factor.

CHAPTER 8

VASCULITIS

Two specific forms of vasculitis that warrant separate consideration are temporal (giant cell or cranial) arteritis and the Takayasu-Ohnishi disease. In addition, there are a miscellany of cases that are not so easily categorized into clinical syndromes.

TEMPORAL ARTERITIS

Temporal arteritis is a widespread arterial inflammation that affects persons in the 60 to 80 year range (occasionally in the 50's) and runs a chronic course of two to three years. The term by which it is traditionally known is poor because many arteries other than the temporal are involved.[120, 312] However, equally untenable are the alternative suggestions of *cranial arteritis* and *giant cell arteritis* because the vascular disease is neither limited to the cranium nor exclusively of the giant cell type.

The proposal[463] that it be named Rumbold's disease has much appeal. This was the name of the first patient to be recognized with the disease. Reported by Jonathan Hutchinson, the patient was described as an 80 year old gentleman's servant, in the family of a peer of the realm, who developed "red streaks on his head." These turned out to be inflamed and swollen temporal arteries.

The prime ophthalmic symptom of temporal arteritis, occurring in approximately one half of all cases,[463, 664] is blindness in one eye, to be followed in one to two weeks by blindness in the opposite eye. The blindness is sometimes preceded by transient blackouts and may be characterized by either an altitudinal hemianopia or complete blindness. As with ischemic optic neuropathy, the blindness is irreversible. The fundus shows typically disc swelling and pallor (Fig. 107), and rarely retinal artery occlusion.[120, 131, 449] Ocular motor palsies occur occasionally.[205, 463]

132

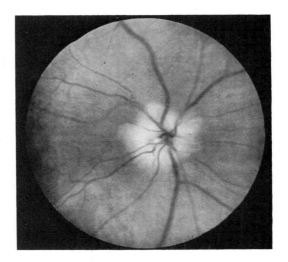

Figure 107 Edema and pallor of the nerve head with temporal arteritis.

The patient was a 77 year old woman who awoke blind in the eye pictured here. Associated symptoms were occipital headache, scalp tenderness, discomfort on chewing, and general malaise. The sedimentation rate was 38 (Westergren). Biopsy of the temporal artery revealed giant cell arteritis.

An occult form of temporal arteritis occurs in which the patient develops the signs of ischemic optic neuropathy with, at that time, no other overt evidence of the disease.[128, 275, 599] This is, in fact, a common mode of presentation.[128] Failure to recognize it is easy, but it is tragic when the opportunity to recognize it at an early stage has been lost.

Because it is treatable, temporal arteritis should be suspected in all cases of ischemic optic neuropathy or retinal artery occlusion in the older age group. Suggestive of the diagnosis are tenderness, nodularity, and loss of pulsation in the temporal arteries; headache[463]; pain or intermittent claudication of the jaw on chewing[335]; fever; malaise; and a history of recent polymyalgia rheumatica[156, 197, 282] (or arthritis[283]). Especially important for diagnosis and for therapeutic regulation is the sedimentation rate. This is invariably elevated during the active stages of the disease. Temporal artery biopsy is diagnostic when positive and should be done in all questionable cases.

A perennially plaguing question is the significance of a negative temporal artery biopsy. Does this rule out a giant cell arteritis in other vessels? The question cannot be answered definitively in our present state of ignorance.

On microscopy the arteries show inflammation in all layers with focal necrosis of the muscularis[544] and local bulging of the wall. The elastica is severely fragmented and giant cells accumulate, sometimes in abundance, along the zone of the previous elastic lamina. Some elastic fragments may be found within the giant cells. The cases in which the ocular and orbital structures have been available for histopathologic study have shown a similar arteritis in the posterior ciliary arteries and in the central artery of the optic nerve.[82, 120, 125, 128, 131, 268, 312, 407, 442, 449, 577, 620, 696] That the retinal arteries usually show no involvement is not surprising since they normally lack an internal elastic lamina and appreciable muscularis. However, it is surprising that the choroidal arteries have so rarely been involved.[131, 696]

Temporal arteritis responds to steroid therapy but this may have to be given in large doses and for long periods of time.[57, 330, 463, 483, 559] The myalgia and malaise respond promptly to steroids but the blindness is irreversible. The ophthalmic importance of steroid treatment is prevention of visual loss. Although blindness has occurred despite treatment,[463] there is substantial inferential evidence that steroids are generally prophylactic. Long-term follow-up requires calibrating the steroid dosage with sedimentation rate.

TAKAYASU-OHNISHI DISEASE

This is a widespread inflammatory arteritis that is especially prone to involve the aorta and its major branches[497, 629]; hence it is included with the pulseless diseases. It occurs most frequently in young Oriental women.[316, 589] The symptoms are the same as those of the aortic arch syndrome and include severe postural vertigo, amaurosis fugax,[230] necrosis of the nasal septum, and ischemic retinopathy.[500, 527] The first ophthalmic signs are low retinal artery pressure and decreased electroretinographic response.[296] Eventually wreathlike arteriovenous anastomoses about the disc may become prominent (Fig. 108).[77, 570, 629] Cataracts often develop along with iris atrophy. Fever, leukocytosis, and an elevated sedimentation rate corroborate the inflammatory etiology.

Pathologically the arteries in the Takayasu-Ohnishi disease show mild inflammation of all the coats with fragmentation of the elastica,

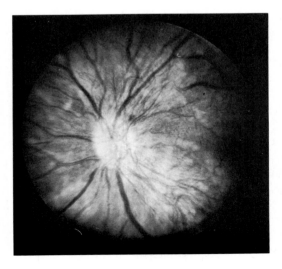

Figure 108 Proliferative retinopathy in the Takayasu-Ohnishi disease.

The patient was a 27 year old Oriental woman with postural amaurosis and hemiplegia. Her brachial pulses were unobtainable.

giant cell reaction, and thrombotic occlusion of the aortic arch and carotid arteries.[209] The eyes show ischemic retinopathy. The cause of the disease is obscure.

MISCELLANEOUS

Nonspecific retinal vasculitis incorporates a spectrum with arbitrary cutoff points at either end. At one extreme is the infiltration of the vessel wall that may occur in any irritable eye. At the other end is the severe inflammatory retinopathy that involves the vessels secondarily. In between are the primary vascular processes in which the inflammation involves, or seems to involve, the vessels primarily. These latter will be a phlebitis when the vein is involved, an arteritis when the artery is involved, and a vasculitis when either or both are involved.

Primary

Since the etiology of the primary vasculitides is practically always obscure, we can classify them only according to their severity, but with the full knowledge that we may be observing a heterogeneous group of entities.[101]

MILD. This form is characterized by mild to moderate congestion of the veins, a few scattered hemorrhages, and swelling of the disc (Fig. 109). It has been variously called "retinal vasculitis"[441] and "papillophlebitis."[437] It occurs predominantly in young persons, perhaps most especially in males, and runs a benign course of several weeks or months. Vision is reduced little, if at all, and several asymptomatic cases have been discovered fortuitously on routine examina-

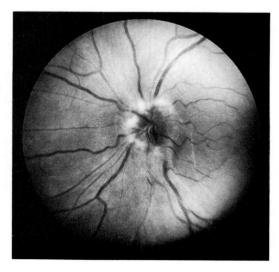

Figure 109 Mild vasculitis. Noteworthy is the swelling of the disc with a corona of exudate (?) and congestion of the vessels.

The patient was a 36 year old man who had mild ocular discomfort and slight reduction in vision with the present eye. The condition subsequently resolved.

tion. Fluoroangiography merely reflects the reduction in perfusion resulting from the elevated venous pressure.[292] The actual evidence that this is an inflammatory process can only be inferred, for all that one sees is venous congestion, nor is there significant elevation of the sedimentation rate, fever, or other evidence of inflammation. Isolated instances have occurred with lupus erythematosus and nonspecific vasculitis elsewhere.[101]

MODERATE. The venous congestion and hemorrhages in this group are more marked than in the previous group and vision is reduced to at least 20/70 (Fig. 110). In contrast to those in the mild group which are unilateral, those in the moderate group are usually bilateral and affect the arteries as well as the veins. The vessels often show focal areas of infiltrate and leakage by fluoroangiography (Fig. 111). The etiology of the moderate variety is as obscure as it is for the mild cases, although isolated instances have been associated with syphilis, arthritis, and post-vaccination. The bilaterality causes confusion with increased intracranial pressure and on occasion craniotomy has been done on mistaken premises.

SEVERE. In this group the fundus shows such extensive hemorrhages as to suggest venous occlusion but the arteries are also involved as indicated by white lines replacing them. The eye may be to-

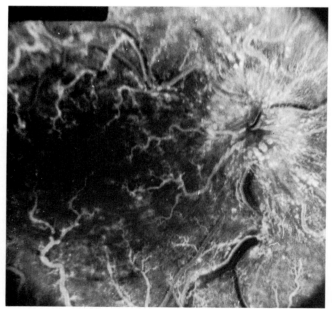

Figure 110   Fluoroangiogram (early phase) with moderate vasculitis. Noteworthy are the dilation of vessels and the diffuse leakage about the optic disc.

The patient was a 27 year old man whose only complaint was moderate reduction in vision. No systemic abnormality was discovered and the condition resolved completely.

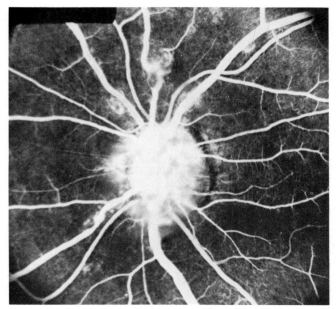

Figure 111 Fluoroangiogram in a patient with moderate vasculitis and systemic sarcoidosis. Noteworthy is the leakage of dye from the disc and along some of the vessels.

The patient is a 50 year old woman with a past history of syphilis and at present a lymphadenopathy due to sarcoid.

tally blind. Such cases may be unilateral or bilateral. The few cases which have become available for histopathology have shown cellular infiltration of the vessels,[435] fibrinoid necrosis of the walls, and massive increase in basement membrane formation.[101] The vein has been found to be thrombosed behind the lamina cribrosa (Fig. 112).

Although no one systemic condition occurs regularly with these severe cases, individual instances have been associated with polyarteritis,[190, 313, 376] Behçet's disease, multiple sclerosis, and granulomatous arteritis elsewhere in the body. Herpes simplex may be a common cause[269] but it is difficult to prove.

The frequent symmetry in the two eyes suggests an allergic angiitis. Injection of homologous, or bovine, retina with Freund's adjuvant into monkeys has produced a retinal periphlebitis[426, 660, 661] but it also produces a uveitis unlike the human cases.

Secondary

Secondary vasculitis is that which occurs with etiologically or clinically distinctive entities and takes various forms.

Toxoplasmosis is a relatively common form of chorioretinal inflammation in which the vessels may be incidentally involved. During

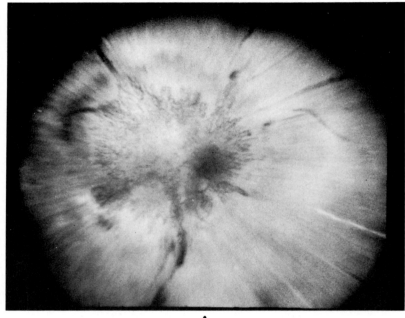

A

Figure 112 Fundus photograph and histopathologic section from an eye with retinal vasculitis. The massive hemorrhages and vascular proliferation point to venous occlusion while the white arteries (combined with total blindness) point to arterial occlusion.

The patient was a 25 year old man who developed persistent pain in the eye and a blurring of vision that progressed to total blindness over a period of several weeks. The etiology was never ascertained but glaucoma ensued and the eye was enucleated on account of pain. The sections show the massive proliferation of vessels on the nerve head and perivascular infiltration of the vessels within the nerve substance.

(Illustration continued on opposite page.)

its active stage the typical toxoplasmic lesion consists of a yellowish mass with overlying fine vitreous opacities. In the ultimate stage of scarring, it consists of a focal scar in which pigment and white tissue replace the normally orange background. The overlying or proximal vessels may show ensheathing and occasionally occlusions but at no time is the vasculitis a conspicuous part of the process. The inflammation may be recurrent but only rarely is the acquired form associated with fever, arthralgia, or other systemic symptoms. The congenital form, however, resulting from infection of the fetus by the mother is often associated with central nervous system involvement.

Cytomegalic inclusion disease produces a secondary vasculitis similar to that produced by toxoplasmosis[115] and may similarly be congenital or acquired. It also occurs with the lymphomas, especially in persons on antimetabolite therapy, and may account for the retinal vasculitis that has been reported with Hodgkin's disease.[516]

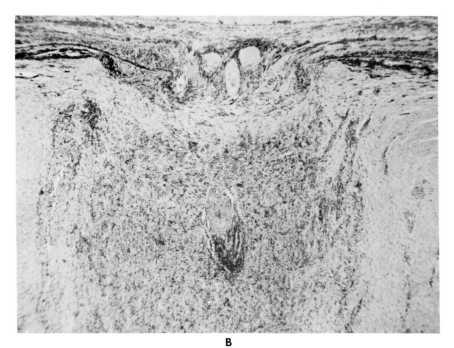

B

Figure 112 Continued.

Behçet's disease is a syndrome characterized by severe retinitis, retinal vasculitis, hypopyon iritis, aphthous ulcers of the mouth and genitalia, fever, arthritis, and erythema nodosum. It is recurrent and eventually fatal with involvement of the central nervous system. The etiology is uncertain but the vasculitis (both arteries and veins) is a conspicuous component.[195, 584, 589] Males are especially prone to the disease and the majority of cases have occurred in Orientals.[586]

A form of peripheral retinitis with a decided vascular component is that which has been variously termed peripheral uveitis, cyclitis, peripheral periphlebitis, and pars planitis. It is a clinical syndrome with white deposits (likened to snow banks) in the far periphery and on the pars plana of the ciliary body, perivenular ensheathing, occasional arterial and venous occlusion,[68] and papilledema. It may be unilateral or bilateral and affects young adults preferentially. Its etiology is unknown.

Sarcoidosis affects the retina and retinal vessels relatively frequently.[6, 115, 264, 665, 704] Especially characteristic are fluffy white deposits on the retina and along retinal vessels appearing in a manner that has been likened to candle wax drippings.[93, 212] The deposits may also occur in the vitreous where their appearance has been likened to snowballs.[421] A more direct involvement of the vessels occurs with the occasional sarcoidosis of the nerve head.[255, 429]

These white conglomerates consist of round cells and epithelioid cells. They often accompany perivascular ensheathing and suggest, therefore, a type of sarcoid periphlebitis.

Eales' disease is usually included among the vasculitides and is commonly believed to have a tuberculous etiology. The evidence for an inflammatory reaction and the assumption of a tuberculous origin are, however, unconvincing. It has therefore been included with the primarily occlusive vasculopathies (p. 116).

SUMMARY

Two types of vasculitis that have been characterized sufficiently to warrant separate identification are temporal arteritis and the Takayasu-Ohnishi syndrome. In addition, there are many other less well-classified vasculitides.

Temporal arteritis (Rumbold's disease) is a systemic vasculitis that classically involves the temporal arteries and frequently causes blindness through involvement of the posterior ciliary arteries and nerve head. It affects the older age group and is often associated with systemic symptoms but may be occult. Elevation of the sedimentation rate significantly distinguishes it from other forms of ischemic optic neuropathy. Histopathologic examination of the temporal arteries, which may be easily biopsied, reveals typically a giant cell arteritis. The ciliary arteries which have become available in postmortem specimens have shown a similar arteritis. Steroids are relatively effective in prevention of visual loss and are dramatically effective in relief of other symptoms of temporal arteritis.

The Takayasu-Ohnishi disease is also a giant cell arteritis but affects primarily young Oriental women. The primary symptoms are those of hypotension attributable to occlusion of the aortic arch vessels. Postural blackouts are early manifestations. The retinal arterial pressure is characteristically low and the retinal vessels proliferate from the nerve head to form a characteristic peripapillary wreath. Cataracts result from the ischemia of the eye.

Several less well-identified types of retinal vasculitis with obscure etiologies are divided for convenience into mild, moderate, and severe. The mild type simply simulates venous congestion with little or no visual disturbance. The moderate type may involve both arteries and veins with variable effects on vision. The severe type produces massive hemorrhagic and exudative reactions with, on pathologic examination, necrotizing arteritis.

In addition, vasculitis occurs nonspecifically with various inflammatory lesions of the retina and choroid. It may thus be a secondary feature of toxoplasmosis, cytomegalic inclusion disease, Behçet's disease, peripheral uveitis, and sarcoidosis.

CHAPTER 9

NEURO-OPHTHALMIC COMPLICATIONS OF INTRACRANIAL VASCULAR DISEASE

Much of neuro-ophthalmology revolves about vascular disease. The signs and symptoms conveniently divide themselves into those involving the motor system, manifesting disturbances of eye movement, and those of the sensory system, manifesting disturbances in visual acuity and visual fields.

OCULAR MOTOR SYSTEM

Vascular disease may affect the peripheral ocular motor nerves, the internuclear connections in the brain stem, or any of the centers for conjugate gaze. The manifestations provide conveniently localizable signs.

Peripheral Nerve Paralysis

Paralysis of the sixth cranial nerve (abducens) results in inability to abduct the eye. In consequence, the patient is cross-eyed in the primary position of gaze and habitually turns his head to the opposite side for binocular vision (Fig. 113). Paralysis of the fourth cranial nerve (trochlear) results in inability to intort the eye or to turn the eye downward when it is adducted. Characteristic is the compensatory head tilt to the opposite shoulder (Fig. 114). Paralysis of the third cranial nerve (oculomotor) involves all the other ocular muscles with consequent inability to turn the eye up, down, or in, together with ptosis of the lid and nonreactive mydriasis of the pupil (Fig. 115).

141

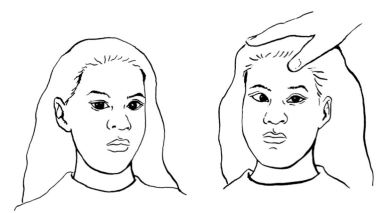

Figure 113   Left-sided sixth nerve paralysis. The patient obtains binocular vision by turning her head to the left so that both eyes are conjugately turned to the right. When the patient is asked to look to the left (and head is forcibly turned to the right), the left eye does not rotate past the midline, with consequent severe esotropia.

Lesions of the ocular motor nerves can be caused by many lesions of which aneurysms, diabetes, and trauma provide the most common vasculopathies.

ANEURYSMS.   The common berry or saccular aneurysms occur chiefly at the bifurcations of the major intracranial arteries and produce topical symptoms according to their sites of origin. Some familiarity with the intracranial anatomy of the carotid artery and of the circle of Willis is essential for the understanding of these symptoms (Fig. 116).

The internal carotid artery enters the skull through the carotid canal and passes forward in the cavernous sinus to emerge dorsally at the level of the an-

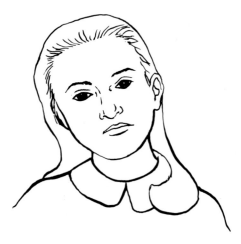

Figure 114   Head tilt with left fourth nerve paralysis. Characteristic is the head tilt toward the right shoulder since, in this position, the left trochlear muscle is normally relaxed. Only in this position will the patient obtain binocular vision.

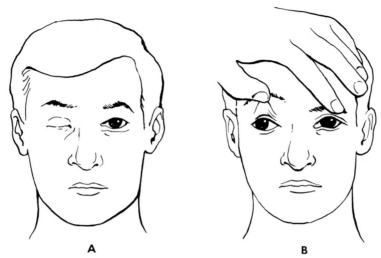

A   **B**

Figure 115 Right-sided third nerve paralysis. Evident are *(A)* complete ptosis due to paralysis of the levator muscle, and *(B)* exodeviation of the eye (seen when the lid is elevated) due to paralysis of the medial rectus muscle.

terior clinoid process. Within the cavernous sinus the carotid artery lies in close apposition to all the ocular motor nerves and to the first two divisions of the trigeminal nerve. Only small arterial branches are given off by the carotid artery within the sinus.

The ophthalmic artery, the first major branch of the carotid within the skull, arises just after the carotid emerges from the cavernous sinus. Two other important branches before terminating in the anterior cerebral and middle cerebral arteries are (1) the anterior choroidal artery supplying the choroidal plexus of the lateral ventricle, parts of the optic tract, and lateral geniculate

Figure 116 Circle of Willis. The major arteries comprising or contributing to this circle are: *A. CEREB.*, anterior cerebral; *IC*, internal carotid; *A. COM.*, anterior communicating; *MC*, middle cerebral; *P. COM.*, posterior communicating; *P. CEREB.*, posterior cerebral; *BA*, basilar artery; *VA*, vertebral artery.

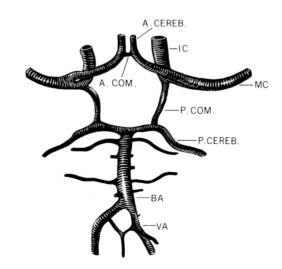

body; and (2) the posterior communicating artery that connects the carotid system with the posterior cerebral system.

While the anterior portion of the circle of Willis and the carotid artery are most intimately associated with the optic nerve, chiasm, and tracts, the posterior portions are especially associated with the ocular motor nerves. Most apt to be involved is the third nerve which passes between the posterior cerebral and superior cerebellar arteries as it emerges from the pons and then comes to lie beneath the posterior communicating artery.

The basilar artery at the base of the pons lies close to the sixth nerves as they emerge from the posterior end of the pons to extend forward over the petrous ridge of the temporal bone.

The saccular aneurysms are best visualized by arteriography and are classified accordingly into infraclinoid and supraclinoid aneurysms. The infraclinoid aneurysms arise from the carotid artery within the cavernous sinus and produce ocular motor palsies,[254] hypesthesia of the first and sometimes of the second division of the trigeminal nerve, a bruit about the eyes, and, when ruptured, a pulsating exophthalmos and congestion of the eye.[462] The supraclinoid aneurysms arise either from the internal carotid artery after its exit from the cavernous sinus or from the circle of Willis. They produce symptoms either by mass compression or by rupture. Aneurysms in the carotid artery or anterior portion of the circle of Willis cause pressure on the optic nerves or tracts (see p. 148), while aneurysms in the posterior portion of the circle cause ocular motor palsies and various neurologic signs. On rupture, the supraclinoid aneurysms produce the characteristic triad of headache, stiff neck, and vomiting, often leading to coma. Papilledema and vitreous hemorrhages are frequently found ophthalmoscopically. The third nerve is most commonly involved but the paralysis, which is due to extension of blood into the nerve trunk, may occur several days before or after the apoplectic episode. Especially characteristic of aneurysms that bleed into the nerve is the combination of sudden pain in and about the eye and a third nerve paralysis. Yet, unlike the infraclinoid aneurysms, trigeminal hypesthesia is absent.

The third nerve paralysis may be permanent or it may resolve two or more months after the onset. With delayed recovery, anomalous eye movements and pupillary reactions result from aberrant regeneration of the nerve fibers.

Aneurysms that rupture within the cavernous sinus cause a cavernous sinus fistula with the syndrome of pulsating exophthalmos, congestion of the conjunctiva, bruit, and ophthalmoplegia. While the diplopia, subjective bruit, and cosmetic blemish are objectionable, the rupture is, unlike its counterpart outside the cavernous sinus, not life-threatening.

It must not be inferred that aneurysms are the sole, or even the most common, cause of cavernous sinus fistulas. Trauma is the usual cause.[444]

Exophthalmos, orbital pain, congestion of the eye, and ophthalmoplegia (especially transient sixth nerve paralysis) also occur with the so-called dural shunt syndromes.[489, 631] This is a type of spontaneous caroto-cavernous fistula that occurs typically in middle-aged women and is due to the development of anomalous connections between the cavernous sinus and terminal branches of either the external or internal carotid artery. The branches most frequently involved are the meningeal branches of the internal maxillary artery from the external carotid system or the meningohypophyseal branches from the internal carotid system. In the former case it is best visualized by arteriography of the external carotid artery.

Included under the heading of aneurysms are the fusiform enlargements of the basilar artery that may at times involve the ocular motor nerves. Although frequently thought to be arteriosclerotic in origin, they probably depend on a congenitally defective wall which results in the compromising dilatation and tortuosity later in life. To differentiate them from true aneurysms, they have been called dolichoectatic arteries.[565]

DIABETES. Diabetes is a relatively common cause of ocular motor paralyses and is especially apt to involve the third nerves. Since it often occurs with pain, it simulates the syndrome caused by aneurysms but differs, usually, in the sparing of the pupil. Several pathologic studies of such nerves have shown a demyelination of the central portions of the nerve in the cavernous sinus[18, 167] or in the subarachnoid space.[671] The pupillary fibers are believed to traverse the peripheral portion of the nerve and thereby be spared. Whether the pathogenesis represents a diabetic mononeuropathy or a vasculopathy has not been decided but the condition resolves, almost invariably, within two months' time without residua.

Internuclear Ophthalmoplegia

That tract in the brain stem connecting the centers for conjugate horizontal gaze with the oculomotor nuclei is the medial longitudinal fasciculus. It is an internuclear tract since it lies between the third nerve nuclei anteriorly and sixth nerve nuclei posteriorly. Lesions of it cause a selective paralysis of adduction on attempted conjugate gaze to one side. Adduction on convergence, however, is often retained. The paralysis, combined with horizontal nystagmus of the abducting eye on lateral gaze and vertical nystagmus of both eyes on up gaze, is called internuclear ophthalmoplegia.

Bilateral internuclear ophthalmoplegia is characteristic of multiple sclerosis, whereas unilateral internuclear ophthalmoplegia is characteristic of vascular lesions in the pons. The latter occurs precipitously with vertigo and various brain stem signs. Pathologic specimens have shown infarcts corresponding to small branches of the basilar artery with discrete involvement of one of the paired medial longitudinal fasciculi.

Conjugate Gaze Paralysis

The cerebral centers for conjugate horizontal gaze are situated in the pre-rolandic frontal area mediating movements of volition and in the occipital area mediating movements of pursuit (the optokinetic response). Stimulation of either area results in deviation of both eyes to the contralateral side. Lesions of these areas result in deviation of the eyes to the homolateral side but this effect is transient and lasts only as long as the patient is stuporous.

The brain stem centers for conjugate horizontal movements are situated in the floor of the fourth ventricle and mediate movements to the homolateral side. Lesions cause a deviation of the eyes to the opposite side which, unlike that due to lesions of cerebral origin, persists. Bilateral lesions cause paralysis of gaze to both sides but retention of full vertical movements.

Conjugate vertical movements are represented in the cerebrum along with the horizontal movements, but in the brain stem they are separated. Whereas horizontal movements are represented posteriorly in the region of the fourth ventricle, vertical movements are represented anteriorly in the mid-brain. Anterior lesions cause a selective paralysis of up gaze and less frequently of down gaze. Such a paralysis together with convergence paralysis and areflexic pupils is called Parinaud's syndrome. It occurs with vascular accidents, trauma, neoplasia (especially pinealomas), or demyelinative diseases.

Nystagmus

Nystagmus comprises oscillations of the eyes that are characteristically rhythmic. It has a wide-ranging pathogenesis that relates more to the site of the lesion than to the etiology. Thus, while it is a common symptom of intracranial vasculopathy it has no particular relevance to vascular disease. The following is, therefore, a very general discussion of nystagmus.

The direction of nystagmus—that is, whether it is horizontal, vertical, or rotary—has prime significance. Also noteworthy are the character of the movements, the duration, and the associated neurologic symptoms.

Congenital nystagmus is typically horizontal. One form, congenital sensory nystagmus, results from poor vision and has movements that in some fields of gaze are pendular. Another form, congenital motor nystagmus, results from a genetic defect in the ocular tracking mechanism and has movements that are jerklike with a fast component toward the side of gaze. The vision in this type is normal or near normal.

Acquired horizontal nystagmus is most characteristic of brain stem lesions and is jerklike with the quick component toward the side of the lesion. It is thus frequent with vascular lesions in the pons whether they be intrinsic or secondary effects of cerebellar lesions. As the lesions progress, the nystagmus becomes progressively coarser until it eventually merges into a frank gaze paresis. Cerebral lesions, on the other hand, are not necessarily accompanied by nystagmus.

Aquired vertical nystagmus is characteristic of posterior fossa lesions whether they be primarily in the brain stem or in the cerebellum. The nystagmus is usually of the upbeat variety, evoked most readily by directing the gaze upward. The less common downbeat nystagmus, evoked by directing the gaze downward, suggests a lesion in the most caudal portion of the brain stem.

Rotary nystagmus indicates involvement of the vestibular mechanism whether this be in the peripheral end-organ and nerve or in the centers of the brain stem. It is usually combined with horizontal nystagmus when of peripheral origin and with both horizontal and vertical nystagmus when of central origin.

Convergence nystagmus, or nystagmus retractorius, is an infrequent form in which the eyes converge rhythmically or retract into the orbit rhythmically on attempted upward gaze.[610] This is usually associated with Parinaud's syndrome (p. 146) and points to a lesion, including vascular accidents, in the roof of the mid-brain.

SENSORY SYSTEM

Localization of Lesions and Symptoms

CHIASM AND ADJACENT VISUAL PATHWAYS.   The optic nerves enter the skull at the most anteromedial portions of the middle cranial fossa and promptly divide in the chiasm. Fibers from each nasal half of one retina cross over to join the uncrossed fibers from the other retina. They then proceed posteriorly in the optic tracts to terminate either in the lateral geniculate body (for the visual fibers) or in the pretectal nuclei (for the pupillary fibers).

Lesions of the chiasm cause bitemporal hemianopic defects in which the central field may or may not be affected. Reduction in visual acuity suggests that some of the non-decussating fibers are also involved. The most common causes of bitemporal hemianopia are pituitary tumors, craniopharyngiomas, and suprasellar meningiomas in that order. Less common causes are aneurysms, vascular accidents, trauma, and pituitary apoplexy. Recognition of bitemporal hemianopia and identification of its cause are vitally important since the chiasmal area is otherwise a neurologically silent area. Roentgenography is indicated in all cases but even this may be unrevealing.[334] Surgical exploration of the chiasmal region is often necessary in doubtful cases.

Lesions of the optic nerve may cause various constrictions of the visual field but are especially apt to cause central scotomas. This vulnerability of the central fibers in the optic nerve has not been satisfactorily explained. Lesions of the optic tract cause a homonymous hemianopia that by itself is not distinguishable from lesions behind the lateral geniculate body. However, lesions of the optic tract, chiasm, or optic nerve differ from those farther posteriorward in the accompanying optic atrophy and different set of neurologic correlates.

Berry aneurysms in the anterior portion of the circle of Willis are relatively common causes of compressions on the optic nerves, chiasm, and tracts.[355, 357] They may, however, rupture into the optic nerve, producing the clinical syndrome of optic nerve apoplexy.[182] More frequently, involvement of the optic nerve produces a central scotoma, an altitudinal hemianopia, or complete blindness. Such aneurysms arise from either the anterior communicating artery (which courses dorsal to the optic nerve) or the anterior cerebral artery and can be mistaken clinically for tumor or optic neuritis. Said to be suggestive of an underlying aneurysm are a fluctuation in symptoms, pain, and ocular motor palsy.[462] Rarely, optic nerve compression results from dolichoectatic basilar arteries.[565]

Aneurysms may compress the optic chiasm, sometimes occupying the sella turcica, and then produce a symptomatic facsimile of a pituitary tumor. These compressive aneurysms arise chiefly from the middle cerebral and posterior communicating arteries and produce a hemianopia that may be confused with that of intracerebral lesions. Arteriography is, of course, the essential means of differentiation.

An alleged lesion is the pressure of sclerosed carotid arteries against the lateral portion of the chiasm or of the optic nerves, causing irregular binasal field defects,[461] but this has not been convincingly demonstrated.[669]

OCCIPITAL.   The occipital lobes are the primary visual centers in the cerebrum, receiving fibers from the lateral geniculate body by way of the visual radiation and making connections with association centers in the more anterior portions of the brain. The calcarine fissure on the medial wall of the occiput is a landmark for representation of vision. The peripheral retina is represented most anteriorly along the calcarine fissure while the macular retina, on which most acute vision depends, is represented posteriorly. Moreover, the upper and lower portions of the retina, divided by the horizontal raphe, are represented above and below the calcarine fissure, respectively. The interhemispheric fissure corresponds to the vertical meridian of the retina, with each hemisphere corresponding to the contralateral visual field.

The arterial supply to the occiput derives almost entirely from the posterior cerebral arteries. These are in turn the terminal divisions of the basilar artery[682] and give off secondary branches to the brain stem and (by way of the thalamogeniculate branch) to the lateral geniculate body and internal capsule. The posterior cerebral circulation is readily accessible for arteriographic study.[343]

Occlusion of the posterior cerebral artery may thus give rise to a variety of signs and symptoms in addition to hemianopia. On the other hand, occlusion of the most distal portions of the posterior cerebral arteries will cause visual defects without other neurologic symptoms, what might be called the silent hemianopias. Moreover, isolated upper and lower quadrantic field defects may result from lesions demarcated by the calcarine fissure.

Several anatomic anomalies are noteworthy. Especially common is the origin of one posterior cerebral artery from the carotid rather than from the basilar system. This may be confusing when vertebral arteriograms fail to demonstrate the "posterior cerebral artery" on one side.

Another significant anomaly is the origin of the ophthalmic artery from the middle meningeal rather than from the carotid artery.

From the viewpoint of the visual changes one can say categorically that homonymous paracentral scotomas that come to the point of fixation (Fig. 117) are pathognomonic of lesions at the posterior pole of the occiput, whereas simple constriction of the field with sparing of the central area is characteristic of the more anterior lesions that affect the visual radiation (Fig. 118).

Bilateral occlusion of the posterior cerebral arteries usually causes complete blindness, although central vision is sometimes spared. This occasional sparing is apparently due to collateral circulation from the choroidal, pericallosal, middle cerebral, and pial vessels.

Serial angiography, combined with magnification and subtraction techniques, is of great value in identifying vascular lesions in the occiput.[343] Occlusion of an entire posterior cerebral artery is infrequently seen, presum-

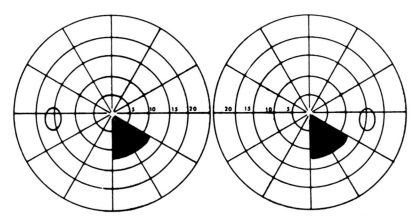

Figure 117 Homonymous paracentral scotomas. This field abnormality is characteristic of lesions of the contralateral occipital pole.

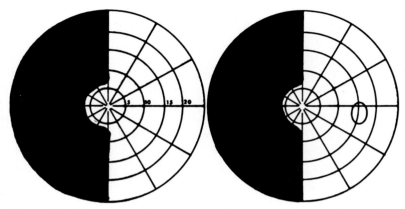

Figure 118   Homonymous hemianopia with sparing of the central area. This field abnormality is characteristic of cerebral lesions anterior to the occipital pole (occipito-parieto-temporal area).

ably because most patients die from concomitant brain stem involvement. Occlusion of its thalamostriate and medial choroidal branches is usually of embolic origin whereas occlusions further along the trunk often result from the pressure of herniation of the hippocampus at the tentorial notch.[354] Whatever the cause of the obstruction of the posterior cerebral artery, retrograde filling by arteriography is an important indication of collateral circulation.

The one most constant symptom of a vascular lesion in the occiput is hemianopia. A normal optokinetic response and the absence of other neurologic signs distinguish the occipital from other cerebral sites. Photopsia (flashes of light) and hallucinations may also occur with occipital vascular lesions and, for some obscure reason, the hallucinations are much more common with lesions in the nondominant hemisphere.

Migraine produces an especially characteristic syndrome that is undoubtedly attributable to vascular disturbances in the occipital lobe. The typical attack of visual migraine begins with scintillating phosphene in one half of the visual field. These scintillations may be amorphous or have picket-fence contours but in either case they are in constant motion and move toward the periphery. Fifteen or so minutes later a hemianopia replaces the scintillations and the patient develops a variably severe headache on the side opposite the visual phenomena. The entire process resolves in a matter of hours but leaves the patient with a "hangover" for a day or so. Variations of this typical pattern are common. The headaches may occur without the scintillations or, in older patients, the visual symptoms may occur without the headaches.[16] Most important is the alternating bilaterality, for this serves as a crucial sign distinguishing migraine from the occipital vascular anomalies which may otherwise simulate it but which involve only one side.

PARIETOTEMPORAL.   The parietotemporal lobes execute most of the integrative functions that serve vision and, most particularly, they relay the visual impulses from the lateral geniculate bodies to the occipital lobes.

The blood supply to the parietotemporal area comes in part from the posterior cerebral artery and its parietotemporal branches but comes chiefly from the middle cerebral and thereby from the carotid system. This contrasts with the occipital lobe, which is supplied by the vertebral-basilar system.

The hemianopia resulting from lesions in the parietotemporal area is homonymous and the field constrictions progress from the periphery toward the center. The defect involves predominantly the lower field with parietal lobe lesions and the upper field with temporal lobe lesions. However, most characteristic of parietotemporal lesions are the associated neurologic symptoms. Lesions in the dominant hemisphere cause alexia and other visual agnosias, along with stereognosia, whereas lesions in the nondominant hemisphere cause constructional apraxia and difficulties in spatial orientation. Also characteristic of parietal lobe lesions is diminution or absence of the optokinetic response on rotation of the field to the side of the lesion, whereas the psychomotor seizures are characteristic of temporal lobe lesions.

Without arteriography it is difficult to distinguish the parietotemporal symptoms of vascular occlusions in the middle cerebral artery from those in the carotid artery. Occlusions of the middle cerebral artery, however, tend to produce symptoms that are abrupt in their onset, whereas those of carotid origin tend to be insidious and progressive.[597] In addition, headache is more conspicuous with carotid disease than with middle cerebral artery disease (possibly owing to the collateral circulation in the carotid system). However, most significant in the differential is, when present, a lower retinal artery pressure on the side of a carotid stenosis.

INTERNAL CAPSULE.   At the posterior end of the internal capsule the entire visual radiation is concentrated in a very small zone. This zone is immediately posterior to the pyramidal fibers to the leg. Hence, relatively small vascular accidents in the posterior end of the internal capsule will cause complete hemianopia and a variable degree of hemiplegia that includes at least the leg muscles.

The blood supply to the internal capsule comes from the lenticulostriate and lenticulo-optic branches of the middle cerebral artery.

In differential diagnosis of hemianopia with vascular lesions in various parts of the brain, the following practical points have been suggested[203]: vascular occlusions in the internal capsule produce complete hemianopia; occlusions in the middle cerebral or carotid artery produce variably complete hemianopia associated with monocular blackouts or blindness on the side of the lesion, motor and sensory signs on the opposite side, convulsions, and aphasia; occlusions of the posterior cerebral artery cause a hemianopia that is also variably complete and associated with vertigo, diplopia, gaze palsies, dysarthria, hearing defects, and staggering gait.

Pathogenesis of Cerebrovascular Accidents Affecting Vision

The majority of cerebrovascular lesions involving the visual system are either embolic or thrombotic. Less common causes are hemorrhage and a variety of functional "steal" syndromes.

The distinction of embolic and thrombotic origins offers clinical problems in which associated systemic conditions are all important. Prior transient ischemic attacks do not necessarily indicate thromboses, as once believed, since small emboli have been found to cause repetitive attacks before a large embolus results in the definitive occlusion (p. 123).

An intracranial vascular accident in a young person with rheumatic heart disease (or with a cardiac myxoma) is presumptive evidence of an embolic origin but in a middle-aged or older person the underlying lesion might be either embolic or thrombotic.

Serial angiography may serve to differentiate embolic and thrombotic occlusions but is most useful in ruling out hemorrhage, aneurysms, neoplasms, and nonvascular lesions of the brain. Most important is the displacement of vessels which occurs with mass lesions but not with vascular occlusions. Narrowing of the vessels does not necessarily point to local disease since it may occur with obstructions downstream.[343] On the other hand, failure of the vessels to fill in the early phase of the angiograms and retrograde filling of the vessels in the late phases points definitely to obstruction with secondary collateral circulation. Occasionally the embolus may be outlined by the contrast substance.[137]

Massive hemorrhage is said to result from rupture of sizable arteries only. It accounts for one quarter of all vascular accidents.[2]

Stenosis of the subclavian artery proximal to its vertebral branch (see Fig. 96, p. 113), or stenosis of the innominate artery proximal to its vertebral branch, produces syndromes that involve the visual system through occipital ischemia.[343, 438, 489, 546] They have been appropriately called the subclavian and innominate "steal" syndromes.[173] Such stenosis causes a low pressure in the homolateral vertebral and brachial arteries. Blood flowing up the opposite vertebral artery is therefore shunted down the homolateral vertebral artery and thence to the arm. It thereby robs the occipital area of blood with resultant hemianopia or blindness.

Although the blackouts or hemianopias usually occur spontaneously, cases have been reported in which use of the hand or posturing of the head will induce transient attacks.

Essential to the diagnosis of the steal syndromes is a disproportionately low blood pressure in the arm of the stenotic side. The retinal blood pressures may be equal or unequal, depending on the coexistent involvement of the carotids. As one might expect, the carotid artery is more apt to be involved with right-sided lesions because of the origin of the carotid from the innominate artery.

As noted previously, aneurysms arise preferentially from the circle of Willis but they may occur along the course of any of the major blood vessels and, by rupture, produce the symptoms of an intracranial vascular accident. There is nothing specific about the hemianopia, and the definitive diagnosis is made only by arteriography. Highly suggestive, however, is a vascular accident occurring in a young person without evident source for emboli and especially when lumbar puncture reveals bloody or xanthomatous spinal fluid.

The aneurysms of the posterior cerebral artery, those which are apt to cause isolated visual defects, have been documented angiographically.[284]

Vascular malformations other than aneurysms may similarly give rise to precipitous symptoms of intracranial vascular accidents but, in comparison with aneurysms, they are more apt to cause intermittent symptoms of phosphene or convulsive episodes.

Classic migraine, which is a common cause of scintillating phosphene and hemianopia, is not known to be associated with any vascular abnormality and differs from the "organic" syndromes in the fluctuations from side to side, the multiplicity of attacks, and the history of familial occurrence. Yet it can easily be mistaken for the symptoms of arteriovenous anomalies, and patients with aneurysms frequently give histories of "migraine."[52]

SUMMARY

Aneurysms of the circle of Willis are a frequent cause of palsies of various ocular motor nerves. Infraclinoid aneurysms arising in the cavernous sinus may produce a total ophthalmoplegia and pulsating exophthalmos or simply a third nerve paralysis and facial hypesthesia. Supraclinoid aneurysms are also apt to produce third nerve paralyses but differ from infraclinoid aneurysms in that they lack the facial hypesthesia and are frequently associated with subarachnoid hemorrhage.

Diabetes is also a relatively frequent cause of paralysis of the third nerve and occasionally of the other ocular motor nerves. As with aneurysms, the onset is often painful but, unlike that with aneurysms, the pupil is typically not dilated.

Internuclear ophthalmoplegia is a syndrome characterized by selective weakness of adduction (that is, of the medial recti) on attempted horizontal gaze. It is due to a lesion in the medial longitudinal fasciculus. Although the bilateral variety is highly suggestive of multiple sclerosis, the unilateral variety points usually to vascular occlusion in the brain stem.

Conjugate gaze palsies (that is, paralysis of the two eyes equally) are due to supranuclear lesions that are often vascular in origin. Lesions in the cerebrum produce, with rare exception, only transient palsies that resolve as the patient regains consciousness, but lesions in the brain stem produce lasting palsies. Those in the pontine region affect horizontal movements, whereas those in the tectal region affect vertical movements.

Nystagmus refers to rhythmic oscillations of the eyes resulting from loss of tone of the conjugate gaze mechanisms. A pendular or sensory variety occurs with congenitally poor vision, whereas a jerk or motor type occurs with lesions anywhere in the nervous system but most conspicuously with brain stem lesions.

The chiasm is the site of decussation of visual fibers from each nasal half of the retina. Lesions of the chiasm, therefore, produce a bitemporal hemianopia. Lesions of the optic nerve, by contrast, produce either peripheral field constriction or, most characteristically, central scotomas. The common vascular cause of chiasmal or optic nerve lesions within the cranium is aneurysms.

The occipital lobes, representing the primary cerebral centers for vision, are exclusively supplied by the posterior cerebral arteries. Unilateral occlusions of these arteries give rise to hemianopia and this may be the only neurologic defect. When only the posterior occipital pole is affected, the field defect will be limited to a paracentral scotoma that comes to the point of fixation. Other symptoms of vascular lesions in the occiput are photopsia and, especially with right-sided lesions, hallucinations.

Lesions of the parietotemporal region produce hemianopic defects that initially span the central area. Those on the left (dominant) side of the brain are apt to cause alexia and visual agnosias, whereas those on the right (nondominant) side cause predominant disturbances in spatial orientation. Since the blood supply of the parietotemporal region derives from the middle cerebral artery, its functions reflect particularly abnormalities of the carotid system.

The visual radiation traverses the posterior end of the internal capsule. Vascular lesions in this region, usually attributable to hemorrhage or occlusion of the lenticulostriate artery, cause complete hemianopia along with variable degrees of hemiplegia.

The pathogenesis of these vascular accidents affecting vision is usually thrombotic, embolic, or hemorrhagic. However, functional ischemia may result from several steal syndromes in which blood is drawn from visual centers of stenotic changes in the hemodynamics, and congenital vascular anomalies may underlie any of the vascular accidents. For the differentiation of these possibilities cerebral angiography is crucial.

BIBLIOGRAPHY

1. Ackerman, A. L.: The ocular manifestations of Waldenström's macroglobulinemia and its treatment. Arch. Ophthalmol. 67:701, 1962.
2. Adams, R. D.: Pathology of cerebral vascular diseases. B. Cranial cerebral lesions. *In* Wright, I. S., and Millikan, C. H. (eds.): *Cerebral Vascular Diseases. Transactions of the Second Conference Held under the Auspices of the American Heart Association, Princeton, New Jersey, January 16–18, 1957.* New York, London, Grune and Stratton, 1958.
3. Adelung, J. C.: Zur Genese der Angioid streaks (Knapp). Klin. Monätsbl. Augenheilkd. 119:241, 1951.
4. Agarwal, L. P., Chhabra, H. N., and Batta, R. K.: Conjunctival vessels in diabetes mellitus. Excerp. Med. Ophthalmol. 21:69, 1967.
5. Albertini, E., Martinesi, L., and Belli, C.: Comparative study of microvessels of the conjunctiva and of other organs. Preliminary note. Excerp. Med. Ophthalmol. 19:110, 1965.
6. Algvere, P.: Fluorescein studies of retinal vasculitis in sarcoidosis. Report of a case. Acta Ophthalmol. (Kbh.) 48:1129, 1970.
7. Allen, R. A., and Straatsma, B. R.: Ocular involvement in leukemia and allied disorders. Arch. Ophthalmol. 66:490, 1961.
8. Amaha, E.: Morphological changes of the bulbar conjunctival vessels. J. Clin. Ophthal. 7:1089, 1959.
9. Amalric, P., and Coscas, G.: Rétinopathie diabétique. I. Angiographie fluorescéinique dans la rétinopathie diabétique, Arch. Ophtalmol. (Paris)27:553, 1967.
10. Anderson, B., Jr., and McIntosh, H. D.: Retinal circulation. Ann. Rev. Med. 18:15, 1967.
11. Anderson, B., Jr., and Saltzman, H. A.: Retinal oxygen utilization measured by hyperbaric blackout. Arch. Ophthalmol. 72:792, 1964.
12. Andersson, B., and Samuelson, A.: Case of hyperglobulinemia with pronounced eye changes and acrocyanosis. Acta Med. Scand. 117:248, 1944.
13. Appelmans, M., and Lamotte, R.: La coagulation sanguine dans les thromboses des veines rétiniennes. Ophthalmologica 129:1, 1955.
14. Appelmans, M., Michiels, J., Mass, J. M., and DeVloo, N.: Ocular manifestations of the dysproteinemias. Arch. Ophthalmol. 22:117, 1962.
15. Aranda, J. V., Saheb, N., Stern, L., and Avery, M. E.: Arterial oxygen tension and retinal vasoconstriction in newborn infants. Am. J. Dis. Child. 122:189, 1971.
16. Aring, C. D.: The migrainous scintillating scotoma. J.A.M.A. 220:519, 1972.
17. Aronson, S. B., II, and Shaw, R.: Corneal crystals in multiple myeloma. Arch. Ophthalmol. 61:541, 1959.
18. Asbury, A. K., Aldredge, H., Hershberg, R., and Fisher, C. M.: Oculomotor palsy in diabetes mellitus: A clinico-pathological study. Brain 93:555, 1970.
19. Ascher, K. W.: Eye manifestations in polycythemia. (Letter). J.A.M.A. 215:295, 1971.
20. Ashby, M., Oakley, B., Lorentz, I., and Scott, D.: Recurrent transient monocular blindness. Br. Med. J. 5362:894, 1963.

155

156 BIBLIOGRAPHY

21. Ashton, N.: Vascular changes in diabetes with particular reference to the retinal vessels. Preliminary report. Br. J. Ophthalmol. 33:407, 1949.
22. Ashton, N.: Injection of the retinal vascular system in the enucleated eye in diabetic retinopathy. Br. J. Ophthalmol. 34:38, 1950.
23. Ashton, N.: Observations on the choroidal circulation. Br. J. Ophthalmol. 36:465, 1952.
24. Ashton, N.: Central areolar choroidal sclerosis: a histo-pathological study. Br. J. Ophthalmol. 37:140, 1953.
25. Ashton, N.: Studies of the retinal capillaries in relation to diabetic and other retinopathies. Br. J. Ophthalmol. 47:521, 1963.
26. Ashton, N.: Ocular changes in multiple myelomatosis. Arch. Ophthalmol. 73:487, 1965.
27. Ashton, N.: Pathophysiology of retinal cotton-wool spots. Br. Med. Bull. 26:143, 1970.
28. Ashton, N., and de Oliveira, F.: Nomenclature of pericytes; intramural and extramural. Br. J. Ophthalmol. 50:119, 1966.
29. Ashton, N., and Harry, J.: The pathology of cotton wool spots and cytoid bodies in hypertensive retinopathy and other diseases. Trans. Ophthalmol. Soc. U.K. 83:91, 1963.
30. Ashton, N., and Henkind, P.: Experimental occlusion of retinal arterioles (using graded glass ballotina). Br. J. Ophthalmol. 49:225, 1965.
31. Ashton, N., Kok, D. A., and Foulds, W. S.: Ocular pathology in macroglobulinaemia. J. Path. Bact. 86:453, 1963.
32. Ashton, N., Pears, M. A., and Pickering, G. W.: Neuroretinopathy following haemorrhage with a discussion on the nature of cytoid bodies. Br. J. Ophthalmol. 45:385, 1961.
33. Ashton, N., Ward, B., and Serpell, G.: Role of oxygen in the genesis of retrolental fibroplasia. A preliminary report. Br. J. Ophthalmol. 37:513, 1953.
34. Ashton, N., Coomes, E. N., Garner, A., and Oliver, D. O.: Retinopathy due to progressive systemic sclerosis. J. Path. Bact. 96:259, 1968.
35. Ashton, N., Dollery, C. T., Henkind, P., Hill, D. W., Paterson, J. W., Ranalho, P. S., and Shakib, M.: Focal retinal ischaemia. Ophthalmoscopic, circulatory and ultrastructural changes. Br. J. Ophthalmol. 50:281, 1966.
36. Ashworth, B.: The electro-oculogram in disorders of the retinal circulation. Am. J. Ophthalmol. 61:505, 1966.
37. Ask-Upmark, E.: On the "pulseless disease" outside of Japan. Acta Med. Scand. 149:161, 1954.
38. Austen, F. K., Carmichael, M. W., and Adams, R. D.: Neurological manifestations of chronic pulmonary insufficiency. N. Engl. J. Med. 257:579, 1957.
39. Babel, J., Gauthier, G., Psilas, K., Ricci, A., Soriano, H., and Tsacopoulos, M.: Les signes oculaires dans les affections carotidiennes. Ophthalmologica 161:324, 1970.
40. Baehr, G.: A diffuse disease of the peripheral circulation (usually associated with lupus erythematosus and endocarditis). Trans. Assoc. Am. Physicians 50:139, 1935.
41. Baghdassarian, S. A., Crawford, J. B., and Rathbun, J. E.: Calcific emboli of the retinal and ciliary arteries. Am. J. Ophthalmol. 69:372, 1970.
42. Ballantyne, A. J.: Retinal changes associated with diabetes and with hypertension. A comparison and contrast. Arch. Ophthalmol. 33:97, 1945.
43. Ballantyne, A. J.: The state of the retina in diabetes mellitus. Trans. Ophthalmol. Soc. U.K. 66:503, 1946.
44. Ballantyne, A. J., and Loewenstein, A.: Diseases of the retina. 1. The pathology of diabetic retinopathy. Trans. Ophthalmol. Soc. U.K. 63:95, 1943.
45. Ballantyne, A. J., and Loewenstein, A.: Retinal micro-aneurysms and punctate haemorrhages. Br. J. Ophthalmol. 28:593, 1944.
46. Ballantyne, A. J., and Michaelson, I. C.: Textbook of the Fundus of the Eye. Edinburgh, Livingstone, 1962.
47. Baum, J. D.: Retinal artery tortuosity in expremature infants. 18 year follow-up on eyes of premature infants. Arch. Dis. Child. 46:247, 1971.
48. Becker, B.: Diabetic retinopathy. Ann. Intern. Med. 37:273, 1952.
49. Becker, B., and Post, L. T.: Retinal vein occlusion; clinical and experimental observations. Am. J. Ophthalmol. 34:677, 1951.

50. Beetham, W. P., Aiello, L. M., Balodimos, M. C., and Koncz, L.: Ruby laser photocoagulation of early diabetic neovascular retinopathy. Preliminary report of a long-term controlled study. Arch. Ophthalmol. 83:261, 1970.
51. Bell, L. G.: Diabetic optic neuropathy. Trans. Ophthalmol. Soc. N.Z. 9:25, 1957.
52. Bergin, J.: Aneurismal and thrombotic lesions of the carotid with ocular presentation. Trans. Ophthalmol. Soc. N.Z. 9:9, 1957.
53. Berlyne, G. M.: Microcrystalline conjunctival calcification in renal failure. A useful clinical sign. Lancet 2:366, 1968.
54. Berneaud-Kötz, G., and Jahnke, K.: Uber einen Fall von ungewöhnlicher Dys- und Paraproteinamie mit auffallenden Augenhintergrundveränderungen (Fundus paraproteinaemicus). Klin. Monätsbl. Augenheilkd. 125:160, 1954.
55. Bernstein, A.: Periarteritis nodosa without peripheral nodules diagnosed antemortem. Am. J. Med. Sci. 190:317, 1935.
56. Birge, H. L.: New theories of vascular disease: with special reference to the syndrome of polycythemia in ocular pathology. Am. J. Ophthalmol. 39:362, 1955.
57. Birkhead, N. C., Wagener, H. P., and Shick, R. M.: Treatment of temporal arteritis with adrenal corticosteroids; results in 55 cases in which lesion was proved at biopsy. J.A.M.A. 163:821, 1957.
58. Bischler, V.: Le fond d'oeil moucheté multicolore manifestation fruste de la maladie de Groenblad et Strandberg. Bull. Mem. Soc. Ophtalmol. 68:287, 1955.
58a. Blau, J. N., and Davis, E.: Small blood vessels in migraine. Lancet 2:740, 1970.
59. Bloodworth, J. M. B., Jr.: Diabetic retinopathy. Diabetes 11:1, 1962.
60. Blumenthal, M., Gitter, K. A., Best, M., and Galin, M. A.: Fluorescein angiography during induced ocular hypertension in man. Am. J. Ophthalmol. 69:39, 1970.
61. Böck, J.: Ein Beitrag zur Periarteriitis nodosa am Auge. Ztschr. F. Augenh. 78:28, 1932.
62. Boeck, J.: Ocular changes in periarteritis nodosa. Am. J. Ophthalmol. 42:567, 1956.
63. Boniuk, M., and Burton, G. L.: Unilateral glaucoma associated with sickle-cell retinopathy. Trans. Am. Acad. Ophthalmol. Otolaryngol. 68:316, 1964.
64. Borgeson, E. J., and Wagener, H. P.: Changes in eye in leukemia. Am. J. Med. Sci. 177:663, 1929.
65. Braendstrup, P.: Central retinal vein thrombosis and hemorrhagic glaucoma. Acta Ophthalmol. Suppl. 35, 1950.
66. Brickner, R. M., and Franklin, C. R.: Visible retinal arteriolar spasm associated with multiple sclerosis; preliminary report. Arch. Neurol. Psychiat. 51:573, 1944.
67. Brihaye-Van Geertruyden, M., Danis, P., and Toussaint, C.: Fundus lesions with disseminated lupus erythematosus. Arch. Ophthalmol. 51:799, 1954.
68. Brockhurst, R. J., Schepens, C. L., and Okamura, I. D.: Uveitis. III. Peripheral uveitis; pathogenesis, etiology and treatment. Am. J. Ophthalmol. 51:19, 1961.
69. Bronner, A., and Lobstein, P. A.: Le syndrome d'occlusion de l'artere ophtalmique. Doc. Ophthalmol. 20:660, 1966.
70. Brotherman, D. P.: Diabetic retinopathy: a perspective. Survey Ophthalmol. 16:359, 1972.
71. Brownstein, S., Font, R. L., and Alper, M. G.: Atheromatous plaques of the retinal blood vessels. Arch. Ophthalmol. 90:49, 1973.
72. Bruce, G. M.: Retinitis in dermatomyositis. Trans. Am. Ophthalmol. Soc. 36:282, 1938.
73. Bullock, J. D., Falter, R. T., Downing, J. E., and Snyder, H. E.: Ischemic ophthalmia secondary to an ophthalmic artery occlusion. Am. J. Ophthalmol. 74:486, 1972.
74. Burian, H. M.: Pigment epithelium changes in arteriosclerotic choroidopathy. Am. J. Ophthalmol. 68:412, 1969.
75. Bürki, Von E.: Ueber die Cystinkrankheit im Kleinkindesalter unter besonderer Berücksichtigung des Augenbefundes. Ophthalmologica 101:18, 1941.
76. Büttner, I.: Uber den Verschluss der Vena centralis retinae. Medizinische 48:1945, 1958.
77. Caccamise, W. C., and Okuda, K.: Takayasu's or pulseless disease. An unusual syndrome with ocular manifestations. Am. J. Ophthalmol. 37:784, 1954.
78. Cagianut, B.: Le syndrome oculaire de la macroglobulinemie (Syndrome de Waldenstrom). Ann. Ocul. (Paris) 191:579, 1958.

79. Caird, F. I.: Diabetic retinopathy as a cause of visual impairment. In *Symposium*, Ref. 254, p. 41.
80. Caird, F. I., Pirie, A., and Ramsell, T. G.: *Diabetes and the Eye*. Oxford, Blackwell Scientific Publications, 1969.
81. Campbell, K.: Intensive oxygen therapy as possible cause of retrolental fibroplasia: clinical approach. Med. J. Aust. 2:48, 1951.
82. Cardell, B. S., and Hanley, T.: A fatal case of giant cell or temporal arteritis. J. Path. Bact. 63:587, 1951.
83. Carlisle, R., Lanphier, E. H., and Rahn, H.: Hyperbaric oxygen and persistence of vision in retinal ischemia. J. Appl. Physiol. 19:914, 1964.
84. Carr, R. E., and Henkind, P.: Retinal findings associated with serum hyperviscosity. Am. J. Ophthalmol. 56:23, 1963.
85. Carr, R. E., and Siegel, I. M.: Electrophysiologic aspects of several retinal diseases. Am. J. Ophthalmol. 58:95, 1964.
86. Carroll, D.: Retinal migraine. Headache 10:9, 1970.
87. Castleman, B.: Case records of the M.G.H. Case 4–1968. N. Engl. J. Med. 278:206, 1968.
88. Chazan, B. I., Balodimos, M. C., Holsclaw, D. S., and Shwachman, H.: Microcirculation in young adults with cystic fibrosis: Retinal and conjunctival vascular changes in relation to diabetes. J. Pediatr. 77:86, 1970.
89. Chazan, B. I., Kuwabara, T., Balodimos, M. C., and Beetham, W. P.: The reactivity and ultrastructure of conjunctival microaneurysms in diabetes. Diabetologia 5:331, 1969.
90. Chester, E. M., and Banker, B. Q.: The role of lipid thrombi in the pathogenesis of diabetic retinopathy. Arch. Intern. Med. 120:397, 1967.
91. Chisholm, J. F.: The progressive changes in the pathology of early retrolental fibroplasia. Am. J. Ophthalmol. 49:1155, 1960.
92. Christiansson, J.: Retinoschisis in an abortive form of retrolental fibroplasia. Acta Ophthalmol. 41:147, 1963.
93. Chumbley, L. C., and Kearns, T. P.: Retinopathy of sarcoidosis. Am. J. Ophthalmol. 73:123, 1972.
94. Coats, G.: Further cases of thrombosis of the central vein. Roy. Lond. Ophthal. Hosp. Rep. 16:516, 1906.
95. Coats, G.: Der Verschluss der Zentralvene der Retina. Eine Übersicht über 36 pathologisch-anatomisch untersuchte Fälle. Albrecht von Graefes Arch. Klin. Ophthalmol. 86:341, 1913.
96. Cogan, D. G.: Blackouts not obviously due to carotid occlusion. Arch. Ophthalmol. 66:180, 1961.
97. Cogan, D. G.: Development and senescence of the human retinal vasculature. Doyne Memorial Lecture, 1963. Trans. Ophthalmol. Soc. U.K. 83:465, 1963.
98. Cogan, D. G.: Diabetic retinopathy. N. Engl. J. Med. 270:787, 1964.
99. Cogan, D. G.: Two views of choroidal angiosclerosis. (Editorial). Arch. Ophthalmol. 73:309, 1965.
100. Cogan, D. G.: *Neurology of the Visual System*. Springfield, Illinois, Charles C Thomas, 1966.
101. Cogan, D. G.: Retinal and papillary vasculitis. *In* Cant, J. Stanley (ed.): *The William MacKenzie Centenary Symposium on the Ocular Circulation in Health and Disease*. St. Louis, C. V. Mosby, 1969.
102. Cogan, D. G.: Visual hallucinations as release phenomena. Albrecht von Graefes Arch. Klin. Ophthalmol. 188:139, 1973.
103. Cogan, D. G.: Unpublished.
104. Cogan, D. G., and Henneman, P. H.: Diffuse calcification of the cornea in hypercalcemia. N. Engl. J. Med. 257:451, 1957.
105. Cogan, D. G., and Kuwabara, T.: Ocular changes in experimental hypercholesteremia. Arch. Ophthalmol. 61:219, 1959.
106. Cogan, D. G., and Kuwabara, T.: Arcus senilis. Its pathology and histochemistry. Arch. Ophthalmol. 61:553, 1959.
107. Cogan, D. G., and Kuwabara, T.: Capillary shunts in the pathogenesis of diabetic retinopathy. Diabetes 12:293, 1963.
108. Cogan, D. G., Albright, F., and Bartter, F. C.: Hypercalcemia and band keratopathy; report of nineteen cases. Arch. Ophthalmol. 40:624, 1948.

109. Cogan, D. G., Kuwabara, T., and Moser, H.: Fat emboli in the retina following angiography. Arch. Ophthalmol. 71:308, 1964.
110. Cogan, D. G., Kuwabara, T., and Moser, H.: Metachromatic leucodystrophy. Ophthalmologica 160:2, 1970.
111. Cogan, D. G., Toussaint, D., and Kuwabara, T.: Retinal vascular patterns. IV. Diabetic retinopathy. Arch. Ophthalmol. 66:366, 1961.
112. Cogan, D. G., Kuwabara, T., Moser, H., and Hazard, G. W.: Retinopathy in a case of Farber's lipogranulomatosis. Arch. Ophthalmol. 75:752, 1966.
113. Cogan, D. G., Kuwabara, T., Kinoshita, J., Sheehan, L., and Merola, L.: Cystinosis in an adult. J.A.M.A. 164:394, 1967.
114. Cogan, D. G., Kuwabara, T., Kinoshita, J., Sudarsky, D., and Ring, H.: Ocular manifestations of systemic cystinosis. Arch. Ophthalmol. 55:36, 1956.
115. Coles, R. S.: Uveitis associated with systemic diseases. Survey Ophthalmol. 8:377, 1963.
116. Collier, R. H.: Experimental embolic ischemia of the choroid. Arch. Ophthalmol. 77:683, 1967.
117. Comer, P. B., and Fred, H. L.: Diagnosis of sickle-cell disease by ophthalmoscopic inspection of the conjunctiva. N. Engl. J. Med. 271:544, 1964.
118. Condon, P. I., and Serjeant, G. R.: Ocular findings in homozygous sickle cell anemia in Jamaica. Am. J. Ophthalmol. 73:533, 1972.
119. Connor, P. J., Jr., Juergens, J. L., Perry, H. O., Hollenhorst, R. W., and Edwards, J. E.: Pseudoxanthoma elasticum and angioid streaks. A review of 106 cases. Am. J. Med. 30:537, 1961.
120. Cooke, W. T., Cloake, P. C. P., Govan, A. D. T., and Colbeck, J. C.: Temporal arteritis: a generalized vascular disease. Q.J. Med. 15:47, 1946.
121. Cordes, F. C.: Retinal ischemia with visual loss. Report of 5 cases. Am. J. Ophthalmol. 45:(Part II) 79, 1958.
122. Coyle, J. T., Frank, P. E., Leonard, A. L., and Weiner, A.: Macroglobulinemia and its effect upon the eye. Arch. Ophthalmol. 65:75, 1961.
123. Crock, G.: Clinical syndromes of anterior segment ischaemia. Trans. Ophthalmol. Soc. U.K. 87:513, 1967.
124. Croll, M., Hardy, W. G., Lindner, D. W., Webster, J. E., and Gurdjian, E. S.: Evaluation of ophthalmodynamometric and angiographic findings in patients with internal carotid artery thrombosis. J. Neurosurg. 17:394, 1960.
125. Crompton, M. R.: The visual changes in temporal (giant-cell) arteritis. Report of a case with autopsy findings. Brain 82:377, 1959.
126. Crowe, R. J., Kohner, E. M., Owen, S. J., and Robinson, D. M.: The retinal vessels in congenital cyanotic heart disease. Med. Biol. Illus. 19:95, 1969.
127. Cullen, J. F.: Ischaemic optic neuropathy. Trans. Ophthalmol. Soc. U.K. 87:759, 1967.
128. Cullen, J. F.: Occult temporal arteritis. A common cause of blindness in old age. Br. J. Ophthalmol. 51:513, 1967.
129. Culler, A. M.: Fundus changes in leukemia. Trans. Am. Ophthalmol. Soc. 49:445, 1951.
130. Dahrling, B. E.: The histopathology of early central retinal artery occlusion. Arch. Ophthalmol. 73:506, 1965.
131. Daicker, B., and Keller, H. H.: Riesenzellarteriitis mit endookulärer Ausbreitung und Hypotonia bulbi dolorosa. Klinisch-pathologischer Bericht. Klin. Monätsbl. Augenheilkd. 158:358, 1971.
132. Daktaravichene, E. I.: Blood flow changes in conjunctival vessels of the eyeball in atherosclerosis. Excerp. Med. Ophthalmol. 24:227, 1970.
133. Danielsen, L., Kobayasi, T., Larsen, H. W., Midtgaard, K., and Christensen, H. E.: Pseudoxanthoma elasticum. A clinico-pathological study. Acta Derm. Venereol. (Stockh.) 50:355, 1970.
134. Danis, P., Brauman, J., and Coppez, P.: Les lesions du fond d'oeil au cours de certaines hyperproteinemies (myelome a cryoglobuline, macroglobulinemie). Acta Ophthalmol. (Kbh.) 33:33, 1955.
135. David, N. J., Klintworth, G. K., Friedberg, S. J., and Dillon, M.: Fatal atheromatous cerebral embolism associated with bright plaques in the retinal arterioles. Neurology (Minneap.) 13:708, 1963.
136. David, N. J., Norton, E. W. C., Gass, J. D., and Sexton, R.: Fluorescein retinography in carotid occlusion. Arch. Neurol. 14:281, 1966.

137. Davis, D. O., Rumbaugh, C. L., and Gilson, J. M.: Angiographic diagnosis of small-vessel cerebral emboli. Acta Radiol. (Diagn.) (Stockh.) 9:264, 1969.
138. Davis, E., and Landau, J.: Micropools in the conjunctiva and nailbed. Excerp. Med. Ophthalmol. 15:236, 1961.
139. Davis, E., and Landau, J.: Conjunctival micropools ("microaneurysms") in clinical arteriosclerosis. Bibl. Anat. 10:385, 1969.
140. Davis, M. D.: Vitreous contraction in proliferative diabetic retinopathy. Arch. Ophthalmol. 74:741, 1965.
141. Davis, M. D.: Natural course of diabetic retinopathy. In Kimura, S. J., and Caygill, W. M. (eds.): Vascular Complications of Diabetes Mellitus with Special Emphasis on Microangiopathy of the Eye. St. Louis, C. V. Mosby, 1967.
142. Davis, M. D., Myers, F. L., Engerman, R. L., de Venecia, G., and Magli, Y. L.: Clinical observations concerning the pathogenesis of diabetic retinopathy. In Symposium, Ref. 254, p. 47.
143. DeLong, S. L., Poley, B. J., and McFarlane, J. R., Jr.: Ocular changes associated with long-term chlorpromazine therapy. Arch. Ophthalmol. 73:611, 1965.
144. Denny-Brown, D.: Symposium on specific methods of treatment; treatment of recurrent cerebrovascular symptoms and question of "vasospasm." Med. Clin. North Am. 35:1457, 1951.
145. Denny-Brown, D.: Recurrent cerebrovascular episodes. Arch. Neurol. 2:194, 1960.
146. De Simone, S., and De Conciliis, U.: Strie angioidi della retina (considerazioni cliniche e patogenetiche). Zentralbl. Ophthalmol. 76:53, 1959.
147. De Venecia, G., and Davis, M. D.: Histology and fluorescein angiography of microaneurysms in diabetes mellitus. Invest. Ophthalmol. 6:554, 1967.
148. DeVoe, A. G.: Ocular fat embolism; a clinical and pathologic report. Arch. Ophthalmol. 43:857, 1950.
149. DiChiro, G.: Ophthalmic arteriography. Radiology 77:948, 1961.
150. Dienst, E. C., and Gartner, S.: Pathologic changes in the eye associated with subacute bacterial endocarditis. Report of five cases with autopsy. Arch. Ophthalmol. 31:198, 1944.
151. Dische, Z.: The glycans of the mammalian lens capsule—A model of basement membranes. In Siperstein, M. D., Colwell, A. R., Sr., and Meyer, K. (eds.): Small Blood Vessel Involvement in Diabetes Mellitus. American Institute of Biological Sciences, Washington, D.C., 1964, p. 201.
152. Ditzel, J.: Conjunctival vascular changes in relation to retinopathy and nephropathy of diabetes mellitus. Excerp. Med. Ophthalmol. 22:152, 1968.
153. Ditzel, J., and Sagild, U.: Morphology and hemodynamic changes in the small blood vessels in diabetes mellitus: II. The degenerative and hemodynamic changes in the bulbar conjunctiva of normotensive diabetics. N. Engl. J. Med. 250:587, 1954.
154. Ditzel, J., and St. Clair, R. W.: Clinical method of photographing smaller blood vessels and circulating blood in bulbar conjunctiva of human subjects. Circulation 10:277, 1954.
155. Ditzel, J., and White, P.: Central retinal vein occlusion in juvenile diabetes; case report with consideration of pathogenic relationship between diabetic retinopathy and retinal vein occlusion. J. Chronic Dis. 3:253, 1956.
156. Dixon, A. St. J., Beardwell, C., Kay, A. K., Wanka, J., and Wong, Y. T.: Polymyalgia rheumatica and temporal arteritis. Ann. Rheum. Dis. 25:203, 1966.
157. Dobree, J. H.: Proliferative diabetic retinopathy. Evolution of the retinal lesions. Br. J. Ophthalmol. 48:637, 1964.
158. Dobree, J. H.: Evolution of lesions in proliferative diabetic retinopathy: An 8 year photographic survey. In Symposium, Ref. 254, p. 55.
159. Dollery, C. T.: Dynamic aspects of the retinal microcirculation. Arch. Ophthalmol. 79:536, 1968.
160. Dollery, C. T., Hill, D. W., and Hodge, J. V.: The response of normal retinal blood vessels to angiotensin and noradrenaline. J. Physiol. (London) 165:500, 1963.
161. Dollery, C. T., Henkind, P., Paterson, J. W., Ramalho, P. S., and Hill, D. W.: Focal retinal ischaemia. Part I. Ophthalmoscopic and circulatory changes in focal retinal ischaemia. Br. J. Ophthalmol. 50:285, 1966.
162. Donaldson, D. D.: Retinopathy with dermatomyositis. (Feature Photo). Arch. Ophthalmol. 74:704, 1965.

163. Donders, P. C.: Eales' Disease. Doc. Ophthalmol. *12*:1, 1958.
164. Donders, P. C. (also on behalf of Imhof, J. W., and Baars, H.): Ophthalmological phenomena in Waldenstrom's disease with cryoglobulinaemia. Ophthalmologica *135*:324, 1958.
165. Dowling, J. E.: Organization of vertebrate retinas. Invest. Ophthalmol. 9:655, 1970.
166. Dowling, J. L., and Smith, T. R.: An ocular study of pulseless disease. Arch. Ophthalmol. *64*:236, 1960.
167. Dreyfus, P. M., Hakim, S., and Adams, R. D.: Diabetic ophthalmoplegia. Arch. Neurol. Psychiat. *77*:337, 1957.
168. Duane, T. D., Behrendt, T., and Field, R. A.: Net vascular pressure ratios in diabetic retinopathy. In *Symposium*, Ref. 254, p. 657.
169. Dufour, R., Rumpf, J., Cuendet, J. F., Rosselot, E., and Deller, M. (eds.): *Vascular Diseases in Ophthalmology.* Basel, S. Karger, 1968.
170. Duke-Elder, S.: *System of Ophthalmology. VII. The Foundations of Ophthalmology: Heredity, Pathology, Diagnosis and Therapeutics.* St. Louis, C. V. Mosby, 1962, p. 439.
171. Eales, H.: Cases of retinal haemorrhage, associated with epistaxis and constipation. Birmingham Med. Rev. *3*:262, 1880.
172. Edington, G. M., and Sarkies, J. W. R.: Two cases of sickle-cell anaemia associated with retinal microaneurysms. Trans. R. Soc. Trop. Med. Hyg. *46*:59, 1952.
173. Editorial: A new vascular syndrome — "The subclavian steal." N. Engl. J. Med. *265*:912, 1961.
174. Elliot, A. J.: Recurrent intraocular hemorrhage in young adults (Eales's disease). A report of 31 cases. Trans. Am. Ophthalmol. Soc. *52*:811, 1954.
175. Elliot, A. J.: Recurrent intra-ocular hemorrhage in young adults (Eales's disease) with continuous subconjunctival therapy with hydrocortisone. Trans. Am. Ophthalmol. Soc. *56*:383, 1958.
176. Elliot, A. J., and Harris, G. S.: The present status of the diagnosis and treatment of periphlebitis retinae (Eales' disease). Canad. J. Ophthalmol. *4*:117, 1969.
177. Elliott, F. A.: The microcirculation of the brain, retina, and bulbar conjunctiva. *In* Wells, R. (ed.): *The Microcirculation in Clinical Medicine.* New York, Academic Press, 1973.
178. Elliott, F. A., and Leonberg, S. C.: The effect of sludge on the arterial wall. *In* Ditzel, J., and Lewis, D. H. (eds.): *Proceedings of the 6th European Conference on Microcirculation, Aalborg, 1970.* Basel, S. Karger, 1971, p. 371.
179. Ellis, C. J., Hamer, D. B., Hunt, R. W., Lever, A. F., Lever, R. S., Peart, W. S., and Walker, S. M.: Medical investigation of retinal vascular occlusion. Br. Med. J. *2*:1093, 1964.
180. Ellis, P. P., and Hamilton, H.: Retrobulbar neuritis in pernicious anemia. Am. J. Ophthalmol. *48*:95, 1959.
181. Ellis, R. A.: Central retinal artery occlusion associated with cryoglobulinemia. Arch. Ophthalmol. *57*:327, 1957.
182. Ellis, W. G., and Albrand, O.: Optic apoplexy. 5th Neuro-ophthal. Path. Symp., March, 1973, Boston
183. Elschnig, A.: Die diagnostische und prognostische Bedeutung der Netzhauterkrankungen bei Nephritis. Wien Med. Wochenschr. *54*:445, 491, 1904.
184. Engerman, R. L.: Personal communication.
185. Engerman, R. L., and Bloodworth, J. M. B., Jr.: Experimental diabetic retinopathy in dogs. Arch. Ophthalmol. *73*:205, 1965.
186. English, F. P., Bell, J. R., and English, K. P.: Conjunctival vascular pathology associated with diabetic lipemia retinalis. Arch. Ophthalmol. *89*:120, 1973.
187. Ennema, M. C., and Zeeman, W. P. C.: Venous occlusions in the retina. Ophthalmologica *126*:328, 1953.
188. Ernest, J. T., and Potts, A. M.: Pathophysiology of the distal portion of the optic nerve. II. Vascular relationships. Am. J. Ophthalmol. *66*:380, 1968.
189. Eskildsen, P.: Cited in Braendstrup, P., Ref. 65.
190. Evans, H.: Periarteritis nodosa with marked eosinophilia. Proc. R. Soc. Med. *37*:40, 1943.
191. Evans, P. J.: Retrolental fibroplasia. Trans. Ophthalmol. Soc. U.K. *71*:613, 1951.
192. Faris, B. M., and Brockhurst, R. J.: Retrolental fibroplasia in the cicatricial stage.

The complication of rhegmatogenous retinal detachment. Arch. Ophthalmol. 82:60, 1969.

193. Farmer, R. G., Cooper, T., and Pascuzzi, C. A.: Cryoglobulinemia. Report of 12 cases with bone marrow findings. Arch. Intern. Med. 106:483, 1960.

194. Feman, S. S., Bartlett, R. E., Roth, A. M., and Foos, R. Y.: Intraocular hemorrhage and blindness associated with systemic anticoagulation. J.A.M.A. 220:1354, 1972.

195. Fenton, R. H., and Easom, H. A.: Behçet's syndrome. A histopathologic study of the eye. Arch. Ophthalmol. 72:71, 1964.

196. Ferrer, O.: Rapid sequence fluorescein retinal angiography photography. Mod. Probl. Ophthalmol. 9:33, 1971.

197. Fessell, W. J., and Pearson, C. M.: Polymyalgia rheumatica and blindness. N. Engl. J. Med. 276:1403, 1967.

198. Fields, W. S., and Lemak, N. A.: Joint study of extracranial arterial occlusion. VII. Subclavian steal. A review of 168 cases. J.A.M.A. 222:1139, 1972.

199. Fields, W. S., Crawford, E. S., and DeBakey, M. E.: Surgical considerations in cerebral arterial insufficiency. Neurology 8:801, 1958.

200. Fink, A. I.: Vascular fine structure changes in the bulbar conjunctiva associated with sickle cell disease. Am. J. Ophthalmol. 69:563, 1970.

201. Fink, A. I., Funahashi, T., Robinson, M., and Watson, R. J.: Conjunctival blood flow in sickle-cell disease. Preliminary report. Arch. Ophthalmol. 66:824, 1961.

202. Fink, A. I., Funahashi, T., Robinson, M., Watson, R. J., and Felix, M.: Conjunctival blood flow in sickle-cell disease. Responses to local stimuli. Trans. Am. Acad. Ophthalmol. Otolaryngol. 68:301, 1964.

203. Fisher, C. M.: "Intermittent cerebral ischemia." In Wright, I. S., and Millikan, C. H. (eds.): Cerebral Vascular Diseases. Transactions of the Second Conference Held under the Auspices of The American Heart Association, Princeton, New Jersey, January 16–18, 1957. New York, Grune & Stratton, 1958.

204. Fisher, C. M.: Observations of the fundus oculi in transient monocular blindness. Neurology 9:333, 1959.

205. Fisher, C. M.: Ocular palsy in temporal arteritis. Minn. Med. 42:1430, 1959.

206. Fisher, M.: Transient monocular blindness associated with hemiplegia. Arch. Ophthalmol. 47:167, 1952.

207. Fisher, M.: Occlusion of carotid arteries; further experiences. Arch. Neurol. Psychiat. 72:187, 1954.

208. Fleming, K. O.: Bulk studies of the retina in diabetic rabbits. Trans. Canad. Ophthalmol. Soc. 13:123, 1950.

209. Font, R. L., and Naumann, G.: Ocular histopathology in pulseless disease. Arch. Ophthalmol. 82:784, 1969.

210. Foulds, W. S.: The ocular manifestations of blood diseases. Trans. Ophthalmol. Soc. U.K. 88:345, 1963.

211. Foulds, W. S., Chisholm, I. A., Stewart, J. B., and Wilson, T. M.: The optic neuropathy of pernicious anemia. Arch. Ophthalmol. 82:427, 1969.

212. Franceschetti, A., and Babel, J.: La chorio-rétinite en "taches de bougie," manifestation de la maladie de Besnier-Boeck. Ophthalmologica 118:701, 1949.

213. Francois, J., and Neetens, A.: Importance clinique de l'angioscopie conjonctivale. Ann. Ocul. (Paris) 200:656, 1967.

214. Frankel, J.: Ophthalmodynamometry: A pilot study. Am. J. Ophthalmol. 52:85, 1961.

215. Frayser, R., Knisely, W. H., Barnes, R., and Satterwhite, W. M., Jr.: In vivo observations on the conjunctival circulation in elderly subjects. J. Gerontol. 19:494, 1964.

216. Frayser, R., Saltzman, H. A., Anderson, B., Jr., Hickam, J. B., and Sieker, H. O.: The effect of hyperbaric oxygenation on retinal circulation. Arch. Ophthalmol. 77:265, 1967.

217. Fredrickson, D. S., Gotto, A. M., and Levy, R. I.: Familial lipoprotein deficiency. (Abetalipoproteinemia, hypobetalipoproteinemia and Tangier disease.) In Stanbury, J. B., Wyngaarden, J. B., and Fredrickson, D. S. (eds.): The Metabolic Basis of Inherited Disease. 3rd ed. New York, McGraw-Hill Book Company, 1972, p. 493.

218. Freedman, B. J.: Papilloedema, optic atrophy and blindness due to emphysema and chronic bronchitis. Br. J. Ophthalmol. 47:290, 1963.

219. Frenkel, M., and Russe, H. P.: Retinal telangiectasia associated with hypogam-maglobulinemia. Am. J. Ophthalmol. *63*:215, 1967.
220. Friedenwald, J. S.: Disease processes versus pictures in interpretation of retinal vascular lesions. Arch. Ophthalmol. *37*:403, 1947.
221. Friedenwald, J. S.: A new approach to some problems of retinal vascular disease. (The Jackson Memorial Lecture.) Am. J. Ophthalmol. *32*:487, 1949.
222. Friedenwald, J. S.: Diabetic retinopathy. The Fourth Francis I. Proctor Lecture. Am. J. Ophthalmol. *33*:1187, 1950.
223. Friedenwald, J. S., and Rones, B.: Ocular lesions in septicemia. Arch. Ophthalmol. *5*:175, 1931.
224. Friedman, E.: Choroidal blood flow; pressure-flow relationships. Arch. Ophthalmol. *83*:95, 1970.
225. Friedman, E., Smith, T. R., and Kuwabara, T.: Retinal microcirculation in vivo. Invest. Ophthalmol. *3*:217, 1964.
226. Friedman, E., Smith, T. R., Kuwabara, T., and Beyer, C. K.: Choroidal vascular patterns in hypertension. Arch. Ophthalmol. *71*:842, 1964.
227. Friedman, M., Rosenman, R. H., and Byers, S.: Serum lipids and conjunctival circulation after fat ingestion in men exhibiting type-A behavior pattern. Circulation *29*:874, 1964.
228. Frisen, L.: Genuine, relative, binasal hemianopia. Report of a case. Acta Ophthalmol. *49*:734, 1971.
229. Fritz, M. H., and Hogan, M. J.: Fat embolization involving the human eye. Am. J. Ophthalmol. *31*:527, 1948.
230. Frøvig, A. G.: Bilateral obliteration of the common carotid artery; thrombangiitis obliterans. Acta Psych. Neurol. Supp. *39*, 1946.
231. Funahashi, T.: Patho-histological studies of capillary vessels in the conjunctiva of diabetics. Excerp. Med. Ophthalmol. *18*:536, 1964.
232. Funahashi, T., and Fink, A. I.: The pathology of the bulbar conjunctiva in diabetes mellitus: I. Microaneurysms. Am. J. Ophthalmol. *55*:504, 1963.
233. Funahashi, T., Fink, A., Robinson, M., and Watson, R. J.: Pathology of conjunctival vessels in sickle-cell disease. A preliminary report. Am. J. Ophthalmol. *57*:713, 1964.
234. Garron, L. K.: Cystinosis. Trans. Am. Acad. Ophthalmol. Otolaryngol. *63*:99, 1959.
235. Gass, J. D. M.: Pathogenesis of disciform detachment of the neuroepithelium. III. Senile disciform macular degeneration. Am. J. Ophthalmol. *63*:617, 1967.
236. Gass, J. D. M.: Acute posterior multifocal placoid pigment epitheliopathy. Arch. Ophthalmol. *80*:177, 1968.
237. Gass, J. D. M.: A fluorescein angiographic study of macular dysfunction secondary to retinal vascular disease. I. Embolic retinal artery obstruction. Arch. Ophthalmol. *80*:535, 1968.
238. Gass, J. D. M., and Norton, E. W. D.: Fluorescein studies of patients with macular edema and papilledema following cataract extraction. Trans. Am. Ophthalmol. Soc. *64*:232, 1966.
239. Gass, J. D. M., and Norton, E. W. D.: Follow-up study of cystoid macular edema following cataract extraction. Trans. Am. Acad. Ophthalmol. Otolaryngol. *73*:665, 1969.
240. Gay, A. J., and Rosenbaum, A. L.: Retinal artery pressure in asymmetric diabetic retinopathy. Arch. Ophthalmol. *75*:758, 1966.
241. Gay, A. J., Goldor, H., and Smith, M.: Chorioretinal vascular occlusions with latex spheres. Invest. Ophthalmol. *3*:647, 1964.
242. Geeraets, W. J., and Guerry, D., III: Clinical observations on conjunctival capillaries with special reference to sickle cell disease. (Preliminary report.) South. Med. J. *53*:949, 1960.
243. Geeraets, W. J., and Guerry, D., III: Elastic tissue degeneration in sickle-cell disease. Am. J. Ophthalmol. *50*:213, 1960.
244. Gepts, W., and Toussaint, D.: Spontaneous diabetes in dogs and cats. A pathological study. Diabetologia *3*:249, 1967.
245. Gibbs, G. E., Wilson, R. B., and Gifford, H.: Glomerulosclerosis in the long-term alloxan diabetic monkey. Diabetes *15*:258, 1966.
246. Gillilan, L. A.: The collateral circulation of the human orbit. Arch. Ophthalmol. *65*:684, 1961.

247. Gills, J. P., Jr., and Paton, D.: Mottled fundus oculi in pseudoxanthoma elasticum. A report on two siblings. Arch. Ophthalmol. *73*:792, 1965.
248. Gitter, K. A., Houser, B. P., Sarin, L. K., and Justice, J., Jr.: Toxemia of pregnancy; an angiographic interpretation of fundus changes. Arch. Ophthalmol. *80*:449, 1968.
249. Givner, I., and Jaffe, N.: Occlusion of the central retinal artery following anesthesia. Arch. Ophthalmol. *43*:197, 1950.
250. Gnad, H. D.: Ein Verfahren zur Fluorescenzkinematographie der menschlichen Netzhaut. Albrecht von Graefes Arch. Klin. Ophthalmol. *182*:82, 1971.
251. Gnad, H. D.: Zur prinzipiellen Möglichkeit der Darstellung der Fluoreszenzangiographie der menschlichen Netzhaut auf dem Fernsehschirm. Klin. Monätsbl. Augenheilkd. *160*:229, 1972.
252. Goldberg, M. F.: Classification and pathogenesis of proliferative sickle retinopathy. Am. J. Ophthalmol. *71*:649, 1971.
253. Goldberg, M. F.: Natural history of untreated proliferative sickle retinopathy. Arch. Ophthalmol. *85*:428, 1971.
254. Goldberg, M. F., and Fine, S. L. (eds.): *Symposium on the Treatment of Diabetic Retinopathy.* Public Health Service Publ. No. 1890. Arlington, Va., U.S. Dept. of Health, Education and Welfare, 1969.
255. Goldberg, M. S., and Newell, F. W.: Sarcoidosis with retinal involvement. Report of two cases. Arch. Ophthalmol. *32*:93, 1944.
256. Goldberg, M. F., Charache, S., and Acacio, I.: Ophthalmologic manifestations of sickle cell thalassemia. Arch. Intern. Med. *128*:33, 1971.
257. Goldberg, M. F., Cotlier, E., Fichenscher, L. G., Kenyon, K., Enat, R., and Borowsky, S. A.: Macular cherry-red spot, corneal clouding, and β-galactosidase deficiency. Arch. Intern. Med. *128*:387, 1971.
258. Goldsmith, J.: Periarteritis nodosa with involvement of the choroidal and retinal arteries. Am. J. Ophthalmol. *29*:435, 1946.
259. Goldstein, I., and Wexler, D.: The ocular pathology of periarteritis nodosa. Arch. Ophthalmol. *2*:288, 1929.
260. Goldstein, I., and Wexler, D.: Bilateral atrophy of the optic nerve in periarteritis nodosa. A microscopic study. Arch. Ophthalmol. *18*:767, 1937.
261. Gomensoro, J. B., Maslenikov, V., Azambuja, N., Fields, W. S., and Lemak, N. A.: Joint study of extracranial arterial occlusion. VIII. Clinical-radiographic correlation of carotid bifurcation lesions in 177 patients with transient cerebral ischemic attacks. J.A.M.A. *224*:985, 1973.
262. Goodman, G., von Sallmann, L., and Holland, M. G.: Ocular manifestations of sickle-cell disease. Arch. Ophthalmol. *58*:655, 1957.
263. Goren, S. B.: Retinal edema secondary to oral contraceptives. Am. J. Ophthalmol. *64*: 447, 1967.
264. Gould, H., and Kaufman, H. E.: Sarcoid of the fundus. Arch. Ophthalmol. *65*:453, 1961.
265. Graham, M. V.: Carotid artery disease. Trans. Ophthalmol. Soc. U.K. *88*:5, 1968.
266. Green, W. R., and Koo, B. S.: Behçet's disease; a report of the ocular histopathology of one case. Survey Ophthalmol. *12*:324, 1967.
267. Green, W. R., Friedman-Kien, A., and Banfield, W. G.: Angioid streaks in Ehlers-Danlos syndrome. Arch. Ophthalmol. *76*:197, 1966.
268. Greenfield, J. C.: Discussion in: Brain, W. R., Pres., Discussion on some less common cerebrovascular diseases. Proc. R. Soc. Med. (Section of Neurology) *44*:855, 1951.
269. Greite, J. H.: Akute, generalisierte transsudative Periphlebitis retinae. Klin. Monätsbl. Augenheilkd. *160*:104, 1972.
270. Griffiths, J. D., Dymock, I. W., Davies, E. W. G., Hill, D. W., and Williams, R.: Occurrence and prevalence of diabetic retinopathy in hemochromatosis. Diabetes *20*:766, 1971.
271. Guerry, D., III, and Wiesinger, H.: Ocular complications in carotid angiography. Am. J. Ophthalmol. *55*:241, 1963.
272. Guest, M. M., Bond, T. P., Cooper, R. G., and Derrick, J. R.: Red blood cells: Change in shape in capillaries. Science *142*:1319, December 6, 1963.
273. Gunn, M.: On ophthalmoscopic evidence of general arterial disease. Trans. Ophthalmol. Soc. U.K. *8*:356, 1897–8.

274. Gunning, A. J., Pickering, G. W., Robb-Smith, A. H. T., and Russell, R. R.: Mural thrombosis of the internal carotid artery and subsequent embolism. Q.J. Med. 33:155, 1964.

275. Gutrecht, J. A.: Occult temporal arteritis. J.A.M.A. 213:1188, 1970.

276. Gyllensten, L. J., and Hellstrom, B. E.: Retrolental fibroplasia—animal experiments; effect of intermittingly administered oxygen on postnatal development of eyes of fullterm mice. Preliminary report. Excerp. Med. Ophthalmol. 8:429, 1954.

277. Haarr, M.: Retinal periphlebitis in multiple sclerosis. Acta Neurol. Scand. (Suppl.) 4:39: 270.

278. Hagedoorn, A.: Angioid streaks. Arch. Ophthalmol. 21:746, 1939.

279. Hager, H.: Die Ophthalmo-Dynamographie als Methode zur Beurteilung des Gehirnkreislaufes. Klin. Monätsbl. Augenheilkd. 142:827, 1963.

280. Haining, W. M.: Diagnostic value of intravenous fluorescein studies. Br. J. Ophthalmol. 50:587, 1966.

281. Haining, W. M., and Lancaster, R. C.: Advanced techniques for fluorescein angiography. Arch. Ophthalmol. 79:10, 1968.

282. Hamrin, B., Jonsson, N., and Landberg, T.: Arteritis in "polymyalgia rheumatica." Lancet 1:397, 1964.

283. Hamrin, B., Jonsson, N., and Landberg, T.: Involvement of large vessels in polymyalgia arteritica. Lancet 1:1193, 1965.

284. Hanafee, W., and Jannetta, P. J.: Aneurysm as a cause of stroke. Am. J. Roentgen. 98:647, 1966.

285. Haney, W. P., and Preston, R. E.: Ocular complications of carotid arteriography in carotid occlusive disease. A report of three cases. Arch. Ophthalmol. 67:127, 1962.

286. Hannon, J. F.: Vitreous hemorrhages associated with sickle cell–hemoglobin C disease. Am. J. Ophthalmol. 42:707, 1956.

287. Hara, M., Hiwatashi, S., Saito, K., Ono, Y., and Suzuki, T.: Electron microscopic study of conjunctival blood vessels of patients with diabetic retinopathy. Excerp. Med. Ophthalmol. 22:228, 1968.

288. Hardenbergh, F. E.: Idiopathic central retinal artery occlusion. Case report and presentation of a general guide to therapy. Arch. Ophthalmol. 67:556, 1962.

289. Harding, F., and Knisely, M. H.: Settling of sludge in human patients. Angiology 9:317, 1958.

290. Harris, L. S., Cohn, K., Toyofuku, H., Lonergan, E., and Galin, M. A.: Conjunctival and corneal calcific deposits in uremic patients. Am. J. Ophthalmol. 72:130, 1971.

291. Harris, W.: The Facial Neuralgias. London, H. Milford, 1937.

292. Hart, C. D., Sanders, M. D., and Miller, S. J. H.: Benign retinal vasculitis; clinical and fluorescein angiographic study. Br. J. Ophthalmol. 55:721, 1971.

293. Hart, C. T., and Haworth, S.: Bilateral common carotid occlusion with hypoxic ocular sequelae. Br. J. Ophthalmol. 55:383, 1971.

294. Hartman, J. D., Young, I., Bank, A. A., and Rosenblatt, S. A.: Fibromuscular hyperplasia of internal carotid arteries. Stroke in a young adult complicated by oral contraceptives. Arch. Neurol. 25:295, 1971.

295. Hausman, L.: Discussion in Wright, I. S., and Millikan, C. H. (eds.): Cerebral Vascular Diseases. Transactions of the Second Conference Held under the Auspices of the American Heart Association, Princeton, New Jersey, January 16–18, 1957. New York and London, Grune and Stratton, 1958, p. 30.

296. Hayashi, H.: Study of pulseless disease and atypical aortitis (Japanese). Excerp. Med. Ophthalmol. 26:168, 1972.

297. Hayreh, S. S.: The central artery of the retina. Its role in the blood supply of the optic nerve. Br. J. Ophthalmol. 47:651, 1963.

298. Hayreh, S. S.: Occlusion of the central retinal vessels. Br. J. Ophthalmol. 49:626, 1965.

299. Hayreh, S. S.: Blood supply of optic nerve head and its role in optic atrophy, glaucoma, and edema of optic disk. Br. J. Ophthalmol. 53:721, 1969.

300. Hayreh, S. S.: Pathogenesis of occlusion of the central retinal vessels. Am. J. Ophthalmol. 72:998, 1971.

301. Hayreh, S. S., and Baines, J. A. B.: Occlusion of the posterior ciliary artery. III. Effects on the optic nerve head. Br. J. Ophthalmol. 56:754, 1972.

302. Hedges, T. R., Jr.: Ophthalmoscopic findings in internal carotid artery occlusion. Am. J. Ophthalmol. 55:1007, 1963.
303. Hedges, T. R.: The aortic arch syndromes. Arch. Ophthalmol. 71:62, 1964.
304. Heisig, N., and Lindner, J.: Vergleich vitalmikroskopischer und histopathologischer Befunde an der terminalen Strombahn bei degenerativen Gefässerkrankungen. Bibl. Anat. 7:530, 1965.
305. Henkes, H. E.: Electroretinography in circulatory disturbances of the retina. II. The electroretinogram in cases of occlusion of the central retinal artery or of one of its branches. Arch. Ophthalmol. 51:42, 1954.
306. Henkind, P.: Ballotini occlusion of retinal arteries. Collateral vessels. Br. J. Ophthalmol. 50:482, 1966.
307. Henkind, P.: Discussion of "chorioretinal vascular occlusions with latex microspheres" (a long term study). Part II. by H. Goldor and A. J. Gay. Invest. Ophthalmol. 6:55, 1967.
308. Henkind, P.: New observations on the radial peripapillary capillaries. Invest. Ophthalmol. 6:103, 1967.
309. Henkind, P.: Radial peripapillary capillaries of the retina. I. Anatomy: human and comparative. Br. J. Ophthalmol. 51:115, 1967.
310. Henkind, P., Charles, N. C., and Pearson, J.: Histopathology of ischemic optic neuropathy. Am. J. Ophthalmol. 69:78, 1970.
311. Henry, M. D., and Chapman, A. Z.: Vitreous hemorrhage and retinopathy associated with sickle-cell disease. Am. J. Ophthalmol. 38:204, 1954.
312. Heptinstall, R. H., Porter, K. A., and Barkley, H.: Giant-cell (temporal) arteritis. J. Path. Bact. 67:507, 1954.
313. Herson, R. N., and Sampson, R.: Ocular manifestations of polyarteritis nodosa. Q.J. Med. 18:123, 1949.
314. Hill, D. W., Dollery, C. T., Hodge, J. V., and Scott, D. J.: Fluorescein studies of the choroidal circulation. Proc. R. Soc. Med. 57:500, 1964.
315. Hiller, H.: Morbus Coats—Miliaraneurysmenretinitis Leber. Klin. Monätsbl. Augenheilkd. 158:225, 1971.
316. Hirose, K.: A study of fundus changes in the early stages of Takayasu-Ohnishi (pulseless) disease. Am. J. Ophthalmol. 55:295, 1963.
317. Hirschboeck, J. S., and Woo, M.: Clinical evaluation of blood "sludge" phenomenon. Am. J. Med. Sci. 219:538, 1950.
318. Hochheimer, B. F.: Angiography of the retina with indocyanine green. Arch. Ophthalmol. 86:564, 1971.
319. Hodge, J. V., Parr, J. C., and Spears, G. F. S.: Comparison of methods of measuring vessel widths on retinal photographs and the effect of fluorescein injection on apparent retinal vessel calibers. Am. J. Ophthalmol. 68:1060, 1969.
320. Hogan, M. J., and Feeney, L.: Electron microscopy of the human choroid. III. The blood vessels. Am. J. Ophthalmol. 51:1084, 1961.
321. Hollenhorst, R. W.: Symposium on diseases of kidney; ophthalmologic aspects of chronic renal disease. Med. Clin. North Am. 35:1023, 1951.
322. Hollenhorst, R. W.: Ocular manifestations of insufficiency or thrombosis of the internal carotid artery. Trans. Am. Ophthalmol. Soc. 56:474, 1958.
323. Hollenhorst, R. W.: Ophthalmodynamometry and intracranial vascular disease. Med. Clin. North Am. 42:951, 1958.
324. Hollenhorst, R. W.: Ocular manifestations of insufficiency or thrombosis of the internal carotid artery. Am. H. Ophthalmol. 47:753, 1959.
325. Hollenhorst, R. W.: The ocular manifestations of internal carotid arterial thrombosis. Med. Clin. North Am. 44:897, 1960.
326. Hollenhorst, R. W.: Significance of bright plaques in the retinal arterioles. J.A.M.A. 178:123, 1961.
327. Hollenhorst, R. W.: Carotid and vertebral-basilar arterial stenosis and occlusion: neuro-ophthalmologic considerations. Trans. Am. Acad. Ophthalmol. Otolaryngol. 66:166, 1962.
328. Hollenhorst, R. W.: The neuro-ophthalmology of strokes. In Smith, J. Lawton (ed.): Neuro-ophthalmology: Symposium of the University of Miami and the Bascom Palmer Eye Institute. Vol. II. St. Louis, C. V. Mosby, 1965.
329. Hollenhorst, R. W., Lensink, E. V., and Whisnant, J. P.: Experimental embolization of the retinal arterioles. Trans. Am. Ophthalmol. Soc. 60:316, 1962.

330. Hollenhorst, R. W., Brown, J. R., Wagener, H. P., and Shick, R. M.: Neurologic aspects of temporal arteritis. Neurology 10:490, 1960.
331. Holley, K. E., Bahn, R. C., McGoon, D. C.: Calcific embolization associated with valvotomy for calcific aortic stenosis. Circulation 28:175, 1963.
332. Holt, J. M., and Gordon-Smith, E. C.: Retinal abnormalities in diseases of the blood. Br. J. Ophthalmol. 53:145, 1969.
333. Honour, A. J., and Russell, R. R.: Intra-arterial embolism in response to injury. Trans. Ophthalmol. Soc. U.K. 81:451, 1961.
334. Horcejada, J., and Salah, S.: Ist de bitemporale Gesichtsfeldausfall an sich eine Indikation zur Chiasmarevision? Wien. Med. Wochenschr. 120:852, 1970.
335. Horton, B.: Headache and intermittent claudication of the jaw in temporal arteritis. Headache 2:29, 1962.
336. Horton, B. T.: Histaminic cephalgia: differential diagnosis and treatment. Proc. Staff Meet. Mayo Clin. 31:325, 1956.
337. Horton, B. T., Magath, T. B., and Brown, G. E.: Undescribed form of arteritis of temporal vessels. Proc. Staff Meet. Mayo Clin. 7:700, 1932.
338. Houser, O. W., and Baker, H. L.: Fibromuscular dysplasia and other uncommon diseases of the cervical carotid artery: Angiographic aspects. Am. J. Roentgenol. Radium Ther. Nucl. Med. 104:201, 1968.
339. Houser, O. W., Baker, H. L., Jr., Sandok, B. A., and Holley, K. E.: Cephalic arterial fibromuscular dysplasia. Radiology 101:605, 1971.
340. Howard, G. M.: Angioid streaks in acromegaly. Am. J. Ophthalmol. 56:137, 1963.
341. Hoyt, W. F.: Some neuro-ophthalmological considerations in cerebral vascular insufficiency. Arch. Ophthalmol. 62:260, 1959.
342. Hoyt, W. F.: Correlative functional anatomy of the optic chiasm. Clin. Neurosurg. 17:189, 1970.
343. Hoyt, W. F., and Newton, T. H.: Angiographic changes with occlusion of arteries that supply the visual cortex. N.Z. Med. J. 72:310, 1970.
344. Huber, A.: Arteriography and phlebography in the diagnosis of orbital affections. Bull. N.Y. Acad. Med. 44:409, 1968.
345. Hughes, B.: The Visual Fields. Oxford, Blackwell Scientific Publications, 1954.
346. Hutchinson, B. T., and Kuwabara, T.: Phosphorylase and uridine diphosphoglucose synthetase in the retina. Arch. Ophthalmol. 68:538, 1962.
347. Immich, H., Jansen, H. H., and Pisani, K.: Die Beziehungen zwischen Arcus lipoides der Hornhaut und Arteriosklerose. Vergleichende Untersuchungen an hand von 500 Sektions-fälle. Klin. Wochenschr. 45:1017, 1967.
348. Irvine, A. R., and Norton, E. W. D.: Photocoagulation for diabetic retinopathy. Am. J. Ophthalmol. 71:437, 1971.
349. Irvine, S. R.: A newly defined vitreous syndrome following cataract surgery; interpreted according to recent concepts of the structure of the vitreous. The Seventh Francis I. Proctor Lecture. Am. J. Ophthalmol. 36:599, 1953.
350. Isaacs, J. P., Swanson, H. S., and Smith, R. A.: Transient childhood strokes from internal carotid stenosis. J.A.M.A. 207:1859, 1969.
351. Jaffe, N. S.: Macular retinopathy after separation of vitreoretinal adherence. Arch. Ophthalmol. 78:585, 1967.
352. Jayle, G. E., Boyer, R. L., and Camo, R. L.: L'Electroretinographie Dynamique en Ophtalmologie. Paris, Masson, 1959.
353. Jedziniak, J. A., and Kinoshita, J. H.: Activators and inhibitors of lens aldose reductase. Invest. Ophthalmol. 10:357, 1971.
354. Jefferson, A., and Sheldon, P.: Transtentorial herniation of the brain as revealed by the displacement of arteries. Acta Radiol. 46:480, 1956.
355. Jefferson, G.: Compression of the chiasma, optic nerves, and optic tracts by intracranial aneurisms. Brain 60:444, 1937.
356. Jefferson, G.: On the saccular aneurysms of the internal carotid artery in the cavernous sinus. Br. J. Surg. 26:267, 1938.
357. Jefferson, G.: Clinical Neurosurgery. Vol. 1. Baltimore, Williams and Wilkins, 1953.
358. Johnson, G. J., and Bloch, K. J.: Immunoglobulin levels in retinal vascular abnormalities and pseudoxanthoma elasticum. Arch. Ophthalmol. 81:322, 1969.
359. Johnson, H. C., and Walker, A. E.: Angiographic diagnosis of spontaneous thrombosis of internal and common carotid arteries. J. Neurosurg. 8:631, 1951.

360. Johnson, W. A., and Kearns, T. P.: Sludging of blood in retinal veins. Am. J. Ophthalmol. *54*:201, 1962.
361. Jorgensen, M. B., and Jorgensen, B. B.: Angiokeratoma corporis diffusum (Fabry). Dan. Med. Bull. *12*:152, 1965.
362. Jütte, A.: Über die Erweiterung der Netzhautvenen bei jugendlischen Diabetikern. *Diabetische Angiopathie*. Berlin, Academie-Verlag, 1964, p. 13.
363. Jütte, L., and Lemke, L.: *Intravitalfärbang am Augenhintergrund mit Fluoreszein-natrium*. Klin. Monätsbl. Augenheilkd. 49, Suppl., 1968.
364. Kahán, A., Kahán, I. L., and Benkó, A.: Erythrocytic anomalies in hereditary vitreo-retinal degeneration (degeneratio hyaloideoretinalis). Br. J. Ophthalmol. *47*:620, 1963.
365. Kahán, A., Kahán, I. L., and Pirityi, K.: Humorale Ursache der Miliaraneurismen-Retinitis (Leber). Klin. Monätsbl. Augenheilkd. *144*:361, 1964.
366. Karjalainen, K.: Occlusion of the central retinal artery and retinal branch arterioles. A clinical, tonographic and fluorescein angiographic study of 175 patients. Acta Ophthalmol. (Kbh.) Suppl. 109, 1971.
367. Karpe, G., Kornerup, T., and Wulfing, B.: The clinical electroretinogram. VIII. The electroretinogram in diabetic retinopathy. Acta Ophthalmol. (Kbh.) *36*:281, 1958.
368. Kearns, T. P.: Fat embolism of the retina demonstrated by a flat retinal preparation. Am. J. Ophthalmol. *41*:1, 1956.
369. Kearns, T. P.: Symposium on hematologic disorders; changes in ocular fundus in blood diseases. Med. Clin. North Am. *40*:1029, 1956.
370. Kearns, T. P., and Hollenhorst, R. W.: Venous-stasis retinopathy of occlusive disease of the carotid artery. Proc. Mayo Clin. *38*:304, 1963.
371. Keith, N. M., Wagener, H. P., and Barker, N. W.: Some different types of essential hypertension: their course and prognosis. Am. J. Med. Sci. *197*:332, 1939.
372. Kennedy, J. E., and Wise, G. N.: Clinicopathological correlation of retinal lesions. Subacute bacterial endocarditis. Arch. Ophthalmol. *74*:658, 1965.
373. Kennedy, J. E., and Wise, G. N.: Retinochoroidal vascular anastomosis in uveitis. Am. J. Ophthalmol. *71*:122, 1971.
374. Kimura, S. J., and Caygill, W. M.: *Vascular Complications of Diabetes Mellitus with Special Emphasis on Microangiopathy of the Eye*. St. Louis, C. V. Mosby, 1967.
375. Kimura, S., and Shirota, N.: Drug-induced thrombocytopenia. A case report of massive bleeding from conjunctiva due to drug-induced thrombocytopenia. Excerp. Med. Ophthalmol. *27*:59, 1973.
376. King, E. F.: Ocular involvement in a case of periarteritis nodosa. Trans. Ophthalmol. Soc. U.K. *55*:246, 1935.
377. Kinsey, V. E.: Retrolental fibroplasia; cooperative study of retrolental fibroplasia and the use of oxygen. Arch. Ophthalmol. *56*:481, 1956.
378. Kirker, G. E. M., and Hausler, H. R.: Effects of hypoxia on the retinal vasculature of the alloxan-diabetic mouse. Can. J. Ophthalmol. *5*:169, 1970.
379. Kirkham, T. H., Wrigley, P. F. M., and Holt, J. M.: Central retinal vein occlusion complicating iron deficiency anaemia. Br. J. Ophthalmol. *55*:777, 1971.
380. Kittel, V.: *Die Biomikroskopie der Bulbusbindehautgefässe des menschen und ihr klinische Verwertbarkeit*. Leipzig, Georg Thieme, 1960.
381. Kleinert, H.: Primäre Netzhautfaltelung im Maculabereich. Albrecht von Graefes Arch. Klin. Ophthalmol. *155*:350, 1954.
382. Klien, B. A.: Obstruction of the central retinal vein. A clinicohistopathologic analysis. Am. J. Ophthalmol. *27*:1339, 1944.
383. Klien, B. A.: Angioid streaks; a clinical and histopathologic study. Am. J. Ophthalmol. *30*:955, 1947.
384. Klien, B. A.: Prevention of retinal venous occlusion. With special reference to ambulatory dicumarol therapy. Am. J. Ophthalmol. *33*:175, 1950.
385. Klien, B. A.: Spontaneous vascular repair; arteriolar and venous cilioretinal communications. Am. J. Ophthalmol. *50*:691, 1960.
386. Klien, B. A.: Comments on the cotton-wool lesion of the retina. Am. J. Ophthalmol. *59*:17, 1965.
387. Klien, B. A.: Sidelights on retinal venous occlusion. Am. J. Ophthalmol. *61*:25, 1966.

388. Klien, B. A.: Ischemic infarcts of the choroid (Elschnig spots). A cause of retinal separation in hypertensive disease with renal insufficiency: a clinical and histopathologic study. Am. J. Ophthalmol. 66:1069, 1968.

389. Klien, B. A., and Olwin, J. H.: A survey of the pathogenesis of retinal venous occlusion; emphasis upon choice of therapy and an analysis of the therapeutic results in fifty-three patients. Arch. Ophthalmol. 56:207, 1956.

390. Knisely, M. H.: Annotated bibliography on sludged blood. Postgrad. Med. 10:15, 1951.

391. Knisely, M. H.: Intravascular erythrocyte aggregation (blood sludge). In Hamilton, W. F., and Dow, P. (eds.): Handbook of Physiology. Section 2: Circulation. Vol. III. Am. Physiol. Soc., Washington, D.C., 1965.

392. Knisely, M. H., Bloch, E. H., Eliot, T. S., and Warner, L.: Sludged blood. Science 106:431, 1947.

393. Knizley, H., Jr., and Noyes, W. D.: Iron deficiency anemia, papilledema, thrombocytosis, and transient hemiparesis. Arch. Intern. Med. 129:483, 1972.

394. Knowles, H. C.: The control of diabetes mellitus and the progression of retinopathy. In Symposium, Ref. 254, p. 115.

395. Knox, D. L.: Ischemic ocular inflammation. Am. J. Ophthalmol. 60:995, 1965.

396. Knox, D. L., and Duke, J. R.: Slowly progressive ischemic optic neuropathy; a clinicopathologic case report. Trans. Am. Acad. Ophthalmol. Otolaryngol. 75:1065, 1971.

397. Koch, H.: Augenveränderungen beim Angiokeratoma universale Fabry. Ber. Dtsch. Ophthalmol. Ges. 55:357, 1949.

398. Kogure, K., David, N. J., Yamanouchi, U., and Choromokos, E.: Infrared absorption angiography of the fundus circulation. Arch. Ophthalmol. 83:209, 1970.

399. Kohner, E. M., and Henkind, P.: Correlation of fluorescein angiogram and retinal digest in diabetic retinopathy. Am. J. Ophthalmol. 69:403, 1970.

400. Kohner, E. M., Dollery, C. T., and Bulpitt, C. J.: Cotton-wool spots in diabetic retinopathy. Diabetes 18:691, 1969.

401. Kohner, E. M., Dollery, C. T., Paterson, J. W., and Oakley, M. B.: Arterial fluorescein studies in diabetic retinopathy. Diabetes 16:1, 1967.

401a. Konrad, R. M., and Zindler, M.: Biomikroskopische Untersuchungen der Konjunktivalgefässe bei Operationen in künstlicher Hypothermie. Anaesthesist 7:307, 1958.

402. Kornerup, T.: Blood pressure and diabetic retinopathy. Acta Ophthalmol. (Kbh.) 35:163, 1957.

403. Kornzweig, A. L., Eliasoph, I., and Feldstein, M.: The retinal vasculature in macular degeneration. Arch. Ophthalmol. 75:326, 1966.

404. Kornzweig, A. L., Eliasoph, I., and Feldstein, M.: Selective atrophy of the radial peripapillary capillaries in chronic glaucoma. Arch. Ophthalmol. 80:697, 1968.

405. Kraus, E., and Lutz, P.: Ocular cystine deposits in an adult. Arch. Ophthalmol. 85:690, 1971.

406. Krayenbuhl, H.: The value of orbital angiography for diagnosis of unilateral exophthalmos. J. Neurosurg. 19:289, 1962.

407. Kreibig, W.: Optikomalazie, die Folge eines Gefässverschlusses im retrobulbaren Abschnitt des Sehnerven. Klin. Monätsbl. Augenheilkd. 122:719, 1953.

408. Kroll, A. J.: Experimental central retinal artery occlusion. Arch. Ophthalmol. 79:453, 1968.

409. Kulvin, S. M., and David, N. J.: Experimental retinal embolism. Arch. Ophthalmol. 78:774, 1967.

410. Kulvin, S. M., Stauffer, L., Kogure, K., and David, N. J.: Fundus angiography in man by intracarotid administration of dye. South. Med. J. 63:998, 1970.

411. Kunkle, E. C., and Anderson, W. B.: Significance of minor eye signs in headache of migraine type. Arch. Ophthalmol. 65:504, 1961.

412. Kuwabara, T., and Aiello, L.: Leukemic miliary nodules in the retina. Arch. Ophthalmol. 72:494, 1964.

413. Kuwabara, T., and Cogan, D. G.: Studies of retinal vascular patterns. 1. Normal architecture. Arch. Ophthalmol. 64:904, 1960.

414. Kuwabara, T., and Cogan, D. G.: Retinal glycogen. Arch. Ophthalmol. 66:680, 1961.

415. Kuwabara, T., and Cogan, D. G.: Retinal vascular patterns. VI. Mural cells of the retinal capillaries. Arch. Ophthalmol. 69:492, 1963.
416. Kuwabara, T., and Cogan, D. G.: Retinal vascular patterns. VII. Acellular change. *In* Bettman, J. W., Chairman: *Symposium on Vascular Disorders of the Eye. Basic Considerations in Anatomy and Physiology.* St. Louis, C. V. Mosby, 1966, p. 77.
417. Kuwabara, T., Carroll, J. M., and Cogan, D. G.: Retinal vascular patterns. Part III. Age, hypertension, absolute glaucoma, injury. Arch. Ophthalmol. 65:708, 1961.
418. Labram, C.: Les micro-anévrismes du champ vasculaire de la conjonctive bulbaire en pathologie interne. Etude biomicroscopique. Ann. Ocul. (Paris) 197:150, 1964.
419. Labram, C., Lestradet, H., and Grégoire, J.: Les micro-anévrysmes des vaisseaux de la conjonctive bulbaire au cours du diabète sucré. Diabete 13:307, 1965.
420. Lack, A., Adolph, W., Ralston, W., Leiby, G., Winsor, T., and Griffith, G.: Biomicroscopy of conjunctival vessels in hypertension. Am. Heart J. 38:654, 1949.
421. Landers, P. H.: Vitreous lesions observed in Boeck's sarcoid. Am. J. Ophthalmol. 32:1740, 1949.
422. LaPiana, F. G., and Penner, R.: Anaphylactoid reaction to intravenously administered fluorescein. Arch. Ophthalmol. 79:161, 1968.
423. Larsen, H.-W.: Photocoagulation in proliferative diabetic retinopathy. A preliminary report. Acta Ophthalmol. (Kbh.) 47:667, 1969.
424. Lauber, H.: Treatment of atrophy of the optic nerve. Arch. Ophthalmol. 16:555, 1936.
425. Lazarow, A., and Speidel, E.: The chemical composition of the glomerular basement membrane and its relationship to the production of diabetic complications. *In* Siperstein, M. D., Colwell, A. R., Sr., and Meyer, K. (eds.): *Small Blood Vessel Involvement in Diabetes Mellitus.* Washington, D.C., American Institute of Biological Sciences, 1964, p. 127.
426. Lerner, E. M., II, Myers, R. E., and von Sallmann, L.: Autoimmune chorioretinitis in rhesus monkeys. Science 162:561, 1968.
427. L'Esperance, F. A., Jr.: The treatment of ophthalmic vascular disease by argon laser photocoagulation. Trans. Am. Acad. Ophthalmol. Otolaryngol. 73:1077, 1969.
428. Levine, R. A., and Henry, M. D.: Ischemic infarction of the retina following carotid angiography. Am. J. Ophthalmol. 55:365, 1963.
429. Levitt, J. M.: Boeck's sarcoid with ocular localization. Survey of the literature and report of a case. Arch. Ophthalmol. 26:358, 1941.
430. Lieb, W. A., Geeraets, W. J., and Guerry, D., III: Sickle-cell retinopathy. Ocular and systemic manifestations of sickle-cell disease. Acta Ophthalmol. (Kbh.), Suppl. 58, 1959.
431. Lindeke, H. I., and Masler, S. R.: Therapy of retinal vein occlusion. Am. J. Ophthalmol. 51:456, 1961.
432. Liversedge, L. A., and Smith, V. H.: Neuromedical and ophthalmic aspects of central retinal artery occlusion. Trans. Ophthalmol. Soc. U.K. 82:571, 1962.
433. Lockhart, G., Von Noorden, G., Dustan, H. P., Corcoran, A. C., and Page, I. H.: The course of retinopathy in treated malignant hypertension. Arch. Intern. Med. 106:205, 1960.
434. Loewenstein, A.: Glomus cells in the human choroid as the basis of arteriovenous anastomoses. Am. J. Ophthalmol. 32:1651, 1949.
435. Loewenstein, A., Michaelson, I. C., and Hill, J.: Retinal vasculitis of the young: a pathological report. Trans. Ophthalmol. Soc. U.K. 66:211, 1946.
436. Lohse, K., and Weller, P.: Die thrombolytische Behandlung akuter Gefässverschlusse in der Ophthalmologie. Klin. Monätsbl. Augenheilkd. 154:167, 1969.
437. Lonn, L. I., and Hoyt, W. F.: Papillophlebitis, a cause of protracted yet benign optic disc edema. Eye Ear Nose Throat Mon. 45:62, 1966.
438. Lord, R. S., Adar, R., and Stein, R. L.: Contribution of the circle of Willis to the subclavian steal syndrome. Circulation 40:871, 1969.
439. Lorentzen, S. E.: Occlusion of the central retinal artery: a follow-up. Acta Ophthalmol. (Kbh.) 47:690, 1969.
440. Luxenberg, M. N., and Mausolf, F. A.: Retinal circulation in the hyperviscosity syndrome. Am. J. Ophthalmol. 70:588, 1970.

441. Lyle, T. K., and Wybar, K.: Retinal vasculitis. Br. J. Ophthalmol. 45:778, 1961.
442. MacFaul, P. A.: Ciliary artery involvement in giant cell arteritis. Br. J. Ophthalmol. 51:505, 1967.
443. MacLean, A. L., and Maumenee, A. E.: Hemangioma of the choroid. Am. J. Ophthalmol. 50:3, 1960.
444. Madsen, P. H.: Carotid-cavernous fistulae. A study of 18 cases. Acta Ophthalmol. (Kbh.) 48:731, 1970.
445. Madsen, P. H.: Ocular findings in 123 patients with proliferative diabetic retinopathy. III. Changes in the posterior segment of the eye. Doc. Ophthalmol. 29:351, 1971.
446. Madsen, P. H.: Pituitary ablation in diabetics with severe retinopathy. Excerp. Med. Ophthalmol. 25:122, 1971.
447. Manschot, W. A.: Subarachnoid hemorrhage: Intraocular symptoms and their pathogenesis. Am. J. Ophthalmol. 38:501, 1954.
448. Manschot, W. A.: Embolism of the central retinal artery originating from an endocardial myxoma. Am. J. Ophthalmol. 48:381, 1959.
449. Manschot, W. A.: A fatal case of temporal arteritis with ocular symptoms. Ophthalmologica 149:121, 1965.
450. Mapstone, R.: Signs of ocular ischaemia. Trans. Ophthalmol. Soc. U.K. 91:231, 1971.
451. Margolis, G.: Hyperbaric oxygenation: the eye as a limiting factor. Science 151:466, 1966.
452. Maroon, J. C., and Campbell, R. L.: Atrial myxoma: a treatable cause of stroke. J. Neurol. Neurosurg. Psychiatry 32:129, 1969.
453. Marshall, J., and Meadows, S.: The natural history of amaurosis fugax. Brain 91:419, 1968.
454. Marshall, R. A.: A review of lesions in the optic fundus in various diseases of the blood. Blood 14:882, 1959.
455. Marx, F.: An arteriographic demonstration of collaterals between internal and external carotid arteries. Acta Radiol. 31:155, 1949.
456. Maumenee, A. E.: Retinal lesions in lupus erythematosus. Am. J. Ophthalmol. 23:971, 1940.
457. Maumenee, A. E.: Fluorescein angiography in the diagnosis and treatment of lesions of the ocular fundus. Trans. Ophthalmol. Soc. U.K. 88:529, 1968.
458. McBrien, D. J., Bradley, R. D., and Ashton, N.: Retinal emboli in stenosis of the internal carotid artery. Lancet 1:697, 1963.
459. McCulloch, C., and Pashby, T. J.: The significance of conjunctival aneurysms in diabetics. Br. J. Ophthalmol. 34:495, 1950.
460. McGee, D. A., McPhedran, R. S., and Hoffman, H. J.: Carotid and vertebral artery disease. Neurology 12:848, 1962.
461. McLean, J. M., and Ray, B. S.: Soft glaucoma and calcification of the internal carotid arteries. Arch. Ophthalmol. 38:154, 1947.
462. Meadows, S. P.: Intracranial aneurysms. In Feiling, A. (ed.): Modern Trends in Neurology. New York, Paul B. Hoeber, 1951.
463. Meadows, S. P.: Temporal or giant cell arteritis. Proc. R. Soc. Med. 59:329, 1966.
464. Mednick, J., Crowther, D., and Hoyt, W. F.: Bilateral cherry-red spots; without clinical cerebral degeneration. Am. J. Ophthalmol. 60:711, 1965.
465. Merin, S., and Freund, M.: Retinopathy in severe anemia. Am. J. Ophthalmol. 66:1102, 1968.
466. Merlen, J. F., Hiltenbrand, C., and Coget, J.: La capillaroscopie au lit de l'ongle et a la conjonctive oculaire dans le diagnostic des acrosyndromes vasculaires. Ann. Cardiol. Angeiol. (Paris) 18:161, 1969.
467. Meyer-Schwickerath, G.: Light Coagulation. (Translated by S. Drance.) St. Louis, C. V. Mosby, 1960.
468. Meyer-Schwickerath, G.: Treatment of diabetic retinopathy with photocoagulation, fluorescein studies. Excerp. Med. Ophthalmol. 25:146, 1971.
469. Meyer-Schwickerath, G., and Schott, K.: Diabetische Retinopathie und Lichtkoagulation. Ophthalmologica Additamentum 158:605, 1969.
470. Michaelson, I. C.: Retinal Circulation in Man and Animals. Springfield, Illinois, Charles C Thomas, 1954.

471. Michaelson, I. C., and Steedman, H. F.: Injection of the retinal vascular system in enucleated eyes. Br. J. Ophthalmol. 33:376, 1949.
472. Michelson, P. E., and Pfaffenbach, D.: Retinal arterial occlusion following ocular trauma in youths with sickle-trait hemoglobinopathy. Am. J. Ophthalmol. 74:494, 1972.
473. Michelson, P. E., Knox, D. L., and Green, W. R.: Ischemic ocular inflammation. Arch. Ophthalmol. 86:274, 1971.
474. Miller, M.: Diabetes associated with acromegaly, hyperadrenocorticism, hemochromatosis, pancreatitis, pancreatectomy and cancer. In Williams, R. H. (ed.): Diabetes. New York, Hoeber, 1960, p. 708.
475. Milletti, M.: Le diagnostic de la thrombose primitive de la carotide interne dans la region cervicale au moyen de la determination des valeurs de la pression systolique de l'artére centrale de la retine. Pressé Med. 54:655, 1946.
476. Millikan, C. H., Siekert, R. G., and Shick, R. M.: Studies in cerebrovascular disease; use of anticoagulant drugs in treatment of intermittent insufficiency of internal carotid arterial system. Proc. Mayo Clin. 30:578, 1955.
477. Minton, J.: Clinical study of 54 cases of occlusion of central artery of retina and its branches. Proc. R. Soc. Med. 30:285, 1937.
478. Mones, R.: Ophthalmodynamometry. J. Mt. Sinai Hosp., New York, 26:71, 1959.
479. Morax, P.-V., and Blanck, C.: A propos de l'utilisation d'un antifongique en pommade associé à un antibiotique et à un corticoide. Bull. Soc. Ophtalmol. Fr. 70:371, 1970.
480. Mörl, H., Fuhrmeister, H., and Ziegan, J.: Klinische manifeste Atherosklerose und Ergebnisse der biomikroskopischen und histologischen Konjunktivaluntersuchung. Angiologica 7:312, 1970.
481. Morris, D. A., and Henkind, P.: Relationship of intracranial, optic-nerve sheath and retinal hemorrhage. Am. J. Ophthalmol. 64:853, 1967.
482. Morse, P. H.: Elschnig's spots and hypertensive choroidopathy. Am. J. Ophthalmol. 66:844, 1968.
483. Mosher, H. A.: The prognosis in temporal arteritis. Arch. Ophthalmol. 62:641, 1959.
484. Mundall, J., Quintero, P., von Kaulla, K. N., Harmon, R., and Austin, J.: Transient monocular blindness and increased platelet aggregability treated with aspirin. A case report. Neurology 22:280, 1972.
485. Mushin, A.: Ocular changes in premature babies receiving controlled oxygen therapy in the neonatal period. Proc. R. Soc. Med. 64:779, 1971.
486. Nanba, K.: Measurement of caliber of retinal blood vessels on fundus photograph. Report I: A method of measurement by Nikon profile projector, especially on magnification. Excerp. Med. Ophthalmol. 26:216, 1972.
487. Nettl, S., Vrcha, L., Sverak, J., and Herout, V.: Pseudotumor cerebri bei Herzpolyp. Schweiz Med. Wochenschr. 87:317, 1957.
488. New, P. F., Price, D. L., and Carter, B.: Cerebral angiography in cardiac myxoma. Correlation of angiographic and histopathological findings. Radiology 96:335, 1970.
489. Newton, T. H., and Hoyt, W. F.: Dural arteriovenous shunts in the region of the cavernous sinus. Neuroradiol. 1:71, 1970.
490. Nicholson, D. H., and Walsh, F. B.: Oral contraceptives and neuro-ophthalmology disorders. J. Reprod. Med. 3:73, 1969.
491. Niesel, P.: Ophthalmodynamometrie. Ophthalmologica 158:342, 1969.
492. Noell, W. K.: Differentiation, metabolic organization, and viability of the visual cell. Arch. Ophthalmol. 60:702, 1958.
493. North, R. R., Fields, W. S., DeBakey, M. E., and Crawford, E. S.: Brachial-basilar insufficiency syndrome. Neurology (Minneap) 12:810, 1962.
494. Nover, A., and Berneaud-Kötz, G.: Experimentelle Untersuchungen über die Permeabilität der Bindehautgefässe. Zugleich ein Beitrag über die Entstehung von Blutyngen bei Paraproteinämien. Albrecht von Graefes Arch. Klin. Ophthalmol. 159:582, 1958.
495. Nover, A., and Berneaud-Kötz, G.: Beobachtungen an den Bindehautgefässen bei der Makroglobulinämie Waldenström. Medizinische 29:1364 and 1367, 1959.
496. Novotny, H. R., and Alvis, D. L.: A method of photographing fluorescence in circulating blood in the human retina. Circulation 24:82, 1961.

497. Ohnishi: Cited by Hirose, K., and Baba, K.: A study of Takayasu-Ohnishi's (pulseless) disease. Am. J. Ophthalmol. 55:554, 1963.
498. Okun, E.: The effectiveness of photocoagulation in the therapy of proliferative diabetic retinopathy (PDR). (A controlled study in 50 patients.) Trans. Am. Acad. Ophthalmol. Otolaryngol. 72:246, 1968.
499. Okun, E., Johnston, G. P., and Bonkuk, I.: *Management of Diabetic Retinopathy; a Stereoscopic Presentation.* St. Louis, C. V. Mosby, 1971.
500. Ostler, H. B.: Pulseless disease (Takayasu's disease). Am. J. Ophthalmol. 43:583, 1957.
501. Owens, W. C., and Owens, E. U.: Retrolental fibroplasia in premature infants. Am. J. Ophthalmol. 32:1, 1949.
502. Pach, J., Dorndof, W., and Ganshirt, H.: Ophthalmodynamographie beim Carotis-verschluss. Z. Neurol. 199:224, 1971.
503. Paris, G. L., and Macoul, K. L.: Reversible bullous retinal detachment in chronic renal disease. Am. J. Ophthalmol. 67:249, 1969.
504. Paterson, J. W., Dollery, C. T., and Ramalho, P. S.: The effects of platelet aggregates on the retinal microcirculation. Bibl. Anat. 9:85, 1967.
505. Paton, D.: Angioid streaks and sickle cell anemia. A report of two cases. Arch. Ophthalmol. 62:852, 1959.
506. Paton, D.: The conjunctival sign of sickle-cell disease. Arch. Ophthalmol. 66:90, 1961.
507. Paton, D.: The conjunctival sign of sickle-cell disease. Further observations. Arch. Ophthalmol. 68:627, 1962.
508. Paton, D.: Angioid streaks and acromegaly. Am. J. Ophthalmol. 56:841, 1963.
509. Paton, D.: *The Relation of Angioid Streaks to Systemic Disease.* Springfield, Illinois, Charles C Thomas, 1972.
510, Patz, A.: Experimental production of retrolental fibroplasia in animals. *In Retrolental Fibroplasia—Role of Oxygen,* Report of the 16th M & R Pediatric Research Conference, New York, 1955.
511. Patz, A.: Symposium: Retrolental fibroplasia (retinopathy of prematurity). Experimental studies. Trans. Am. Acad. Ophthalmol. Otolaryngol. 59:25, 1955.
512. Patz, A.: The role of oxygen in retrolental fibroplasia. Trans. Am. Ophthalmol. Soc. 66:940, 1968.
513. Patz, A., and Maumenee, A. E.: Studies on diabetic retinopathy. I. Retinopathy in a dog with spontaneous diabetes mellitus. Am. J. Ophthalmol. 54:532, 1962.
514. Patz, A., Maumenee, A. E., and Ryan, S. J.: Argon laser photocoagulation, advantages and limitations. Trans. Am. Acad. Ophthalmol. Otolaryngol. 75:569, 1971.
515. Patz, A., Berkow, J. W., Maumenee, A. E., and Cox, J.: Studies on diabetic retinopathy. II. Retinopathy and nephropathy in spontaneous canine diabetes. Diabetes 14:700, 1965.
516. Pau, H.: Phlebitis und Periphlebitis retinae bei Lymphogranulomatose (Hodgkin). Klin. Monätsbl. Augenheilkd. 152:655, 1968.
517. Paufique, L., and Royer, J.: Les signes oculaires des dysproteinemies. Ann. Ocul. (Paris) 192:721, 1959.
518. Pavlou, A. T., and Wolff, H. G.: The bulbar conjunctival vessels in occlusion of the internal carotid artery. Arch. Intern. Med. 104:53, 1959.
519. Pears, M. A., and Pickering, G. W.: Changes in the fundus oculi after haemorrhage. Q.J. Med. 29:153, 1960.
520. Penner, R., and Font, R. L.: Retinal embolism from calcified vegetations of aortic valve. Arch. Ophthalmol. 81:565, 1969.
521. Percival, S. P. B.: Ocular findings in thrombotic thrombocytopenic purpura (Moschcowitz's disease). Br. J. Ophthalmol. 54:73, 1970.
522. Perraut, L. E., and Zimmerman, L. E.: The occurrence of glaucoma following occlusion of the central retinal artery. Arch. Ophthalmol. 61:845, 1959.
523. Petersen, R. A., and Rosenthal, A.: Retinopathy and papilledema in cyanotic congenital heart disease. Pediatrics 49:243, 1972.
524. Peterson, R. D. A., Cooper, M. D., and Good, R. A.: Lymphoid tissue abnormalities associated with ataxia-telangiectasia. Am. J. Med. 41:342, 1966.
525. Pickering, G. W.: *High Blood Pressure.* London, Churchill, 1955.
526. Pinkerton, R. M. H., and Robertson, D. M.: Corneal and conjunctival changes in dysproteinemia. Invest. Ophthalmol. 8:357, 1969.

527. Pinkham, R. A.: The ocular manifestations of the pulseless syndrome. Acta XVIII Concil. Ophthalmol. 1:348, 1954.
528. Pollack, I. P., and Becker, B.: Cytoid bodies of the retina in a patient with scleroderma. Am. J. Ophthalmol. 54:655, 1962.
529. Polychronakos, D. J., and Chryssafis, B.: Die periphere Iridektomie mit skleraler Kauterisation (Scheiesche Operation). Klin. Monätsbl. Augenheilkd. 157:463, 1970.
530. Pope, C. H.: Retinal capillary microaneurysms. A concept of pathogenesis. Diabetes 9:9, 1960.
531. Poulsen, J. E.: Recovery from retinopathy in a case of diabetes with Simmonds' disease. Diabetes 2:7, 1953.
532. Preston, R. E., and Petrohelos, M. A.: Application of ophthalmodynamometry in carotid artery surgery. A report of 26 cases. Am. J. Ophthalmol. 53:806, 1962.
533. Prokop, O., Wabnitz, R.: Vorkommen von Bindehautblutungen bei Lebenden und Toten. Z. Rechtsmed 67:249, 1970.
534. Radnot, M., and Follmann, P.: Rheomacrodex (Dextran) in the treatment of the occlusion of the central retinal vein. Ann. Ophthalmol. 1:58, 1969.
535. Raeder, J. G.: Paratrigeminal paralysis of oculo-pupillary sympathetic. Brain 47:149, 1924.
536. Rahman, A. N.: The ocular manifestations of hereditary dystopic lipidosis (angiokeratoma corporis diffusum universale). Arch. Ophthalmol. 69:708, 1963.
537. Raitta, C.: Der Zentralvenen-und netzhautvenenverschluss. Acta Ophthalmol. (Kbh.) (Suppl.) 83,1965.
538. Raynaud, G., Manent, P., and Bourgeois, H.: Les "hemorragies sous-conjonctivales", leurs rapports avec la fragilité capillaire, leur traitement. Bull. Soc. Ophtalmol. Fr. 68:951, 1968.
539. Reese, A. B.: Symposium: Retrolental fibroplasia (retinopathy of prematurity). Trans. Am. Acad. Ophthalmol. Otolaryngol. 59:39, 1955.
540. Reese, A. B.: Telangiectasis of the retina and Coats' disease. The eleventh Sanford R. Gifford lecture. Am. J. Ophthalmol. 42:1, 1956.
541. Reese, A. B., and McGavic, J. S.: Relation of field contraction to blood pressure in chronic primary glaucoma. Arch. Ophthalmol. 27:845, 1942.
542. Regnault, F., Castany, M. A., and Bregeat, P.: Les vaisseux de la conjonctive chez les diabétiques. Etude clinique et électromicroscopique. Ann. Med. Interne (Paris) 121:519, 1970.
543. Reichling, W.: 2. Embolie in die Zentralarterie und mehrere Gefässe des Zinnschen Gefässkranzes bei Pseudo-myxom des Herzens. Mit 5 Abbildungen im Text. Ber. Deutsch. Ophthalmol. Ges. 50:329, 1934.
544. Reinecke, R. D., and Kuwabara, T.: Temporal arteritis. I. Smooth muscle cell involvement. Arch. Ophthalmol. 82:446, 1969.
545. Reinecke, R. D., Kuwabara, T., Cogan, D. G., and Weis, D. R.: Retinal vascular patterns. Part V: Experimental ischemia of the cat eye. Arch. Ophthalmol. 67:470, 1962.
546. Reivich, M., Holling, E., Roberts, B., and Toole, J. F.: Reversal of blood flow through the vertebral artery and its effect on cerebral circulation. N. Engl. J. Med. 265:878, 1961.
547. Rifkind, B. M.: Corneal arcus and hyperlipoproteinaemia. Survey Ophthalmol. 16:295, 1972.
548. Riley, F. C., Jr., and Moyer, N. J.: Oculosympathetic paresis associated with cluster headaches. Am. J. Ophthalmol. 72:763, 1971.
549. Ring, H. G., and David, N. J.: Experimental air embolism. Arch. Ophthalmol. 81:830, 1969.
550. Rosen, E.: Fundus in pseudoxanthoma elasticum. Am. J. Ophthalmol. 66:236, 1968.
551. Rosen, E.: Vascular malformations in the human retina. Am. J. Ophthalmol. 67:501, 1969.
552. Rosen, E. S.: Fluorescence Photography of the Eye; a Manual of Dynamic Clinical Ocular Fundus Pathology. With contributions by Bryan Ashworth and Sven Järpe. London, Butterworth, 1969.
553. Ross, R. S., and McKusick, V. A.: Aortic arch syndromes. Diminished or absent pulses in arteries arising from arch of aorta. Arch. Intern. Med. 92:701, 1953.

554. Roth, A. M., and Foos, R. Y.: Surface wrinkling retinopathy in eyes enucleated at autopsy. Trans. Am. Acad. Ophthalmol. Otolaryngol. 75:1047, 1971.
555. Rothstein, T.: Bilateral, central retinal vein closure as the initial manifestation of polycythemia. Am. J. Ophthalmol. 74:256, 1972.
556. Rubenstein, R. A., Yanoff, M., and Albert, D. M.: Thrombocytopenia, anemia, and retinal hemorrhage. Am. J. Ophthalmol. 65:435, 1968.
557. Rucker, C. W.: Sheathing of retinal veins in multiple sclerosis. J.A.M.A. 127:970, 1945.
558. Rudd, C., Evans, P. J., and Peeney, A. L. P.: Ocular complications in thalassaemia minor. Br. J. Ophthalmol. 37:353, 1953.
559. Russell, R. W.: Giant-cell arteritis: a review of 35 cases. Q.J. Med. 28:471, 1959.
560. Russell, R. W.: Observations on the retinal blood vessels in monocular blindness. Lancet 2:1422, 1961.
561. Russell, R. W.: The source of retinal emboli. Lancet 2:789, 1968.
562. Russell, R. W., and Cranston, W. I.: Ophthalmodynamometry in carotid artery disease. J. Neurol. Neurosurg. Psychiatry. 24:281, 1961.
563. Russell, R. W., Ffytche, T. J., and Sanders, M. D.: A study of retinal vascular occlusion using fluorescein angiography. Lancet 2:821, 1966.
564. Ryan, S. J., and Goldberg, M. F.: Anterior segment ischemia following scleral buckling in sickle hemoglobinopathy. Am. J. Ophthalmol. 72:35, 1971.
565. Sacks, J. G., and Lindenburg, R.: Dolicho-ectatic intracranial arteries: Symptomatology and pathogenesis of arterial elongation and distention. Johns Hopkins Med. J. 125:95, 1969.
566. Safar, K.: Uber Drucksteigerung im Gefolge der juvenilen Netzhaut-Glaskörper-blutungen und Verschluss der Zentralvene infolge tuberkuloser Phlebitis, nebst Bemerkungen uber die Entstehungsweise der Netzhautgefäss-tuber-kulose. Arch. f. Ophthalmol. 119:624, 1928.
567. Saltzman, H. A., Hart, L., Sieker, H. O., and Duffy, E. J.: Retinal vascular response to hyperbaric oxygenation. J.A.M.A. 191:290, 1965.
568. Sanders, M.: Personal communication.
569. Sanders, M. D., and Hoyt, W. F.: Hypoxic ocular sequelae of carotid-cavernous fistulae. Study of the causes of visual failure before and after neurosurgical treatment in a series of 25 cases. Br. J. Ophthalmol. 53:82, 1969.
570. Sata, T.: Ein seltener Fall von Arterien-Obliteration. Klin. Wochenschr. 17:1154, 1938.
571. Savir, H., and Kurz, O.: Fundus changes in occlusion of the internal carotid artery. Ann. Ophthalmol. 2:622, 1970.
572. Scheinberg, P.: General discussion on ophthalmodynamometry. Second session, May 1, 1960. Neurology 11:107, 1961.
573. Scholz, R. O.: Angioid streaks. Arch. Ophthalmol. 26:677, 1941.
574. Schulze, F., and Tost, M.: Uber Bindehautveranderungen bei Morbus Rendu-Osler. Genetische, klinische, histologische und histotopochemische Unter-suchungen. Klin. Monätsbl. Augenheilkd. 148:653, 1966.
575. Schwab, P. J., Okun, E., and Fahey, J. L.: Reversal of retinopathy in Walden-strom's macroglobulinemia by plasmapheresis. A report of two cases. Arch. Ophthalmol. 64:515, 1960.
576. Scott, D. J., Dollery, C. T., Hill, D. W., Hodge, J. V., and Fraser, R.: Fluorescein studies of the retinal circulation in diabetics. Br. J. Ophthalmol. 47:588, 1963.
577. Seitz, R.: On the pathogenesis of occlusion of the retinal arteries. Ber. Dtsch. Ophthalmol. Ges. 64:321, 1961.
578. Seitz, R.: Die Netzhautgefässe Vergleichende ophthalmoskopische und histo-logische Studien an gesunden und kranken Augen. Buch. Augenartz. 40, 1962.
579. Seitz, R.: The Retinal Vessels; Comparative Ophthalmoscopic and Histologic Studies on Healthy and Diseased Eyes. (Translated by F. C. Blodi.) St. Louis, C. V. Mosby, 1964.
580. Sevel, D., Bristow, J. H., Bank, S., Marks, I., and Jackson, P.: Diabetic retinopathy in chronic pancreatitis. Arch. Ophthalmol. 86:245, 1971.
581. Sevin, R.: Diabetic retinopathy. New pathogenic concepts. Adv. Ophthalmol. 24:315, 1971.
582. Sevin, R., and Cuendet, J. F.: Effets d'une association d'anthocyanosides de myr-tille et de β-carotène sur la résistance capillaire des diabétiques. Ophthalmo-logica 152:109, 1966.

583. Shakib, M., and Ashton, N.: Part II. Ultrastructural changes in focal retinal ischaemia. Br. J. Ophthalmol. 50:325, 1966.
584. A histopathological study on Behçet's disease. Excerp. Med. Ophthalmol. 16:62, 1962.
585. Shikano, S. I.: Pathogenesis of cotton wool spots especially in collagen diseases. (Japanese). Excerp. Med. Ophthalmol. 26:158, 1972.
586. Shikano, S., and Shimizu, K.: Atlas of Fluorescence Fundus Angiography. Tokyo, Igaku Shoin, 1968.
587. Shillito, J., and Rockett, R. X.: Retinal embolism: a complication of carotid endarterectomy. J. Neurosurg. 20:718, 1963.
588. Shimizu, K.: Mottled fundus in association with pseudoxanthoma elasticum. Excerp. Med. Ophthalmol. 16:46, 1962.
589. Shimizu, K.: Fluorescein fundus angiography in Behçet's syndrome. Excerp. Med. Ophthalmol. 25:335, 1971.
590. Shimizu, K., and Sano, K.: Pulseless disease. J. Neuropath. Clin. Neurol. 1:37, 1951.
591. Sibay, T. M., and Hausler, H. R.: Eye findings in two spontaneously diabetic related dogs. Am. J. Ophthalmol. 63:289, 1967.
592. Siegrist, A.: Beitrag zur kenntniss der Arteriosklerose der Augengefässe. IX. Cong. Internat. d'Ophtalmol, Utrecht, 1899, p. 131.
593. Sieker, H. O., and Hickam, J. B.: Normal and impaired retinal vascular reactivity. Circulation 7:79, 1953.
594. Silfverskiold, B. P.: Retinal periphlebitis associated with paraplegia. Arch. Neurol. Psychiatr. 57:351, 1947.
595. Silverberg, H. H.: Roth's spots. Mt. Sinai J. Med. N.Y. 37:77, 1970.
596. Silverman, J., Olwin, J. S., and Graettinger, J. S.: Cardiac myxomas with systemic embolization. Review of the literature and report of a case. Circulation 26:99, 1962.
597. Silverstein, A., and Hollin, S.: Internal carotid vs. middle cerebral artery occlusions. Arch. Neurol. 12:468, 1965.
598. Simmonds, N. T.: Embolus of central retinal artery successfully treated by paracentesis. Am. J. Ophthalmol. 54:1129, 1962.
599. Simmons, R. J., and Cogan, D. G.: Occult temporal arteritis. Arch. Ophthalmol. 68:8, 1962.
600. Simpson, T.: Papilledema with emphysema. Br. Med. J. 2:639, 1948.
601. Singer, G.: Migrating emboli of retinal arteries in thrombocythaemia. Br. J. Ophthalmol. 53:279, 1969.
602. Siperstein, M. D., Norton, W., Unger, R. H., and Madison, L. L.: Muscle capillary basement membrane width in normal, diabetic and prediabetic patients. Trans. Assoc. Am. Physicians 79:330, 1966.
603. Skovborg, F., Nielsen, A. V., Lauritzen, E., and Hartkopp, O.: Diameters of the retinal vessels in diabetic and normal subjects. Diabetes 18:292, 1969.
604. Smith, E. W., and Conley, C. L.: Clinical features of genetic variants of sickle cell disease. Bull. Johns Hopkins Hosp. 94:289, 1954.
605. Smith, J. L.: Unilateral glaucoma in carotid occlusive disease. J.A.M.A. 182:683, 1962.
606. Smith, J. L.: The ophthalmodynamometric carotid compression test. Am. J. Ophthalmol. 56:369, 1963.
607. Smith, J. L., and Cogan, D. G.: The ophthalmodynamometric posture test. Am. J. Ophthalmol. 48:735, 1959.
608. Smith, J. L., Gass, J. D. M., and Justice, J., Jr.: Fluorescein fundus photography of angioid streaks. Br. J. Ophthalmol. 48:517, 1964.
609. Smith, J. L., Zieper, I. H., and Cogan, D. G.: Observations on ophthalmodynamometry. J.A.M.A. 170:1403, 1959.
610. Smith, J. L., Zeiper, I., Gay, A. J., and Cogan, D. G.: Nystagmus retractorius. Arch. Ophthalmol. 62:864, 1959.
611. Smith, M. C., and Hoyt, W. F.: Chronic occlusive disease of the carotid arteries with nondiagnostic or misleading pressures on the retinal arteries. Am. J. Surg. 102:661, 1961.
612. Smith, V. H.: Carotid insufficiency. Trans. Ophthalmol. Soc. U.K. 80:253, 1960.

613. Smith, V. H.: The clinical value of ophthalmodynamometry. Proc. R. Soc. Med. *54*:859, 1961.
614. Soni, K. G., and Woodhouse, D. F.: Retinal vascular occlusion as a presenting feature of glaucoma simplex. Br. J. Ophthalmol. *55*:192, 1971.
615. Sorsby, A., and Crick, R. P.: Central areolar choroidal sclerosis. Br. J. Ophthalmol. *37*:129, 1953.
616. Spalter, H. F.: Abnormal serum proteins and retinal vein thrombosis. Arch. Ophthalmol. *62*:868, 1959.
617. Spalter, H. F.: Ophthalmodynamometry and carotid artery thrombosis. Am. J. Ophthalmol. *47*:453, 1959.
618. Spalter, H. F., TenEick, R. E., and Nahas, G. G.: Effect of hypercapnia on retinal vessel size at constant intracranial pressure. Am. J. Ophthalmol. *57*:741, 1964.
619. Speiser, P., Gittelsohn, A. M., and Patz, A.: Studies on diabetic retinopathy. III. Influence of diabetes on intramural pericytes. Arch. Ophthalmol. *80*:332, 1968.
620. Spencer, W. H., and Hoyt, W. F.: A fatal case of giant-cell arteritis (temporal or cranial arteritis) with ocular involvement. Arch. Ophthalmol. *64*:862, 1960.
621. Stansbury, J. R.: Optic atrophy in diabetes mellitus. A report of three cases in one family. Am. J. Ophthalmol. *31*:1153, 1948.
622. Stein, M. R., and Gay, A. J.: Acute chorioretinal infarction in sickle cell trait. Report of a case. Arch. Ophthalmol. *84*:485, 1970.
623. Stein, M. R., and Parker, C. W.: Reactions following intravenous fluorescein. Am. J. Ophthalmol. *72*:861, 1971.
624. Swash, M., and Earl, C. J.: Transient visual obscurations in chronic rheumatic heart disease. Lancet *2*:323, 1970.
625. Swietliczko, I., and David, N. J.: Fluorescein angiography in experimental ocular hypertension. Am. J. Ophthalmol. *70*:351, 1970.
626. Swietliczko, I., Szapiro, J., and Polis, Z.: Value of retinal artery pressure determination in the diagnosis of internal carotid artery thrombosis. The role of the carotid compression test. Am. J. Ophthalmol. *52*:862, 1961.
627. Sybers, H. D., and Boake, W. C.: Coronary and retinal embolism from left atrial myxoma. Arch. Pathol. *91*:179, 1971.
628. Sykowski, P.: Diabetic retrobulbar neuritis. Am. J. Ophthalmol. *32*:1589, 1949.
629. Takayasu, S.: A case with curious change in the central retinal artery. Acta Soc. Ophthalmol. Jap. *12*:554, 1908.
630. Tanenbaum, H. L., Schepens, C. L., Elzeneiny, I., and Freeman, H. M.: Macular pucker following retinal surgery; a biomicroscopic study. Canad. J. Ophthalmol. *4*:20, 1969.
631. Taniguchi, R. M., Goree, J. A., and Odom, G. L.: Spontaneous carotid-cavernous shunts presenting diagnostic problems. J. Neurosurg. *35*:384, 1971.
632. Tarkkanen, A., Tala, P., Karjalainen, K., and Virkkula, L.: Augenmanifestationen des Aortenbogensyndroms. Zentralbl. Ophthalmol. *99*:455, 1968.
633. Tavatznik, B., and Rabinowitz, D.: Hyperglyceridemia and lipemia retinalis in hypopituitarism. Bull. Johns Hopkins Hosp. *107*:175, 1960.
634. Taylor, E.: Proliferative diabetic retinopathy. Regression of optic disc neovascularization after retinal photocoagulation. Br. J. Ophthalmol. *54*:535, 1970.
635. Taylor, E., and Dobree, J. H.: Proliferative diabetic retinopathy; site and size of initial lesions. Br. J. Ophthalmol. *54*:11, 1970.
636. Terry, T. L.: Extreme prematurity and fibroblastic overgrowth of persistent vascular sheath behind each crystalline lens. I. Preliminary report. Am. J. Ophthalmol. *25*:203, 1942.
637. Thomann, H., and Nover, A.: Über das sludged blood Phänomen (intravasale Erythrozytenballung). Med. Klin. *59*:1153, 1964.
638. Thompson, B. W., Read, R. C., and Campbell, G. S.: Aortic arch syndrome. Arch. Surg. *98*:607, 1969.
639. Topilow, A., and Bisland, T.: Diabetes mellitus as a cause of papillitis. Am. J. Ophthalmol. *35*:855, 1952.
640. Toselli, C., Bertoni, G., Alessio, L., and Mannucci, P. M.: High incidence of thalassaemia in patients with intraocular haemorrhages. Ophthalmologica *157*:343, 1969.
641. Tour, R. L., and Hoyt, W. F.: The syndrome of the aortic arch. Ocular manifesta-

tions of "pulseless disease" and a report of a surgically treated case. Am. J. Ophthalmol. *47*(no. 5, pt. II):35, 1959.

642. Toussaint, D.: *Contribution à l'étude anatomique et clinique de la rétinopathie diabétique chez l'homme et chez l'animal.* Pathologia Europaea, Bruxelles, Presses Académiques Européennes, 1968.

643. Toussaint, D., Kuwabara, T., and Cogan, D. G.: Retinal vascular patterns. Part II. Human retinal vessels studied in three dimensions. Arch. Ophthalmol. *65*:575, 1961.

644. Tripathi, R., and Ashton, N.: Electron microscopical study of Coats' disease. Br. J. Ophthalmol. *55*:289, 1971.

645. Trujillo, M. H., Desenne, J. J., and Pinto, H. B.: Reversible papilledema in iron deficiency anemia. Two cases with normal spinal fluid pressure. Ann. Ophthalmol. *4*:378, 1972.

646. Unsworth, A. C.: Retrolental fibroplasia; a preliminary report. Arch. Ophthalmol. *40*:341, 1948.

647. Van Buskirk, E. M., Lessell, S., and Friedman, E.: Pigmentary epitheliopathy and erythema nodosum. Arch. Ophthalmol. *85*:369, 1971.

648. Vander Werff, T. J., and Phil, D.: The pressure measured in ophthalmodynamometry. Arch. Ophthalmol. *87*:290, 1972.

649. Vannas, S., and Orma, H.: Experience of treating retinal venous occlusion with anticoagulant and antisclerosis therapy. Arch Ophthalmol. *58*:812, 1957.

650. Veirs, E. R.: Periphlebitis retinalis associated with intracranial manifestations. Am. J. Ophthalmol. *31*:168, 1948.

651. Verhoeff, F. H.: Obstruction of the central retinal vein. Arch. Ophthalmol. *36*:1, 1907.

652. Verhoeff, F. H.: Histological findings in a case of angioid streaks. Br. J. Ophthalmol. *32*:531, 1948.

653. Verhoeff, F. H., and Simpson, G. V.: Tubercle within central retinal vein hemorrhagic glaucoma; periphlebitis retinalis in other eye. Arch. Ophthalmol. *24*:645, 1940.

654. Victor, D.: Unpublished.

655. Viefhues, T. K., and Strobel, W.: Zur Klinik der Retinopathie bei Anämien. Klin. Monätsbl. Augenheilkd. *134*:643, 1959.

656. Vignalou, M. P.: L'examen. systématique biomicroscopique des vaisseaux conjonctivaux chez l'enfant diabétique. Bull. Soc. Ophthalmol. Fr. *67*:175, 1967.

657. Vinger, P. F., and Sachs, B. A.: Ocular manifestations of hyperlipoproteinemia. Am. J. Ophthalmol. *70*:563, 1970.

658. Vinijchaikul, K.: Primary arteritis of the aorta and its main branches (Takayasu's arteriopathy). A clinicopathologic autopsy study of 8 cases. Am. J. Med. *43*:15, 1967.

659. Volhard, F.: Die Pathogenese der Retinitis Albuminurica. Zentralbl. Gesamte Ophthalmol. *20*:627, 1929.

660. von Sallmann, L., Myers, R. E., Lerner, E. M., II, and Stone, S. H.: Vasculo-occlusive retinopathy in experimental allergic encephalomyelitis. Arch. Ophthalmol. *78*:112, 1967.

661. von Sallman, L., Meyers, R. E., Stone, S. H., and Lerner, E. M.: Retinal and uveal inflammation in monkeys following inoculation with homologous retinal antigen. Arch. Ophthalmol. *81*:374, 1969.

662. Vrabec, Fr.: Spherical swelling of retinal axons in the aged. Br. J. Ophthalmol. *49*:113, 1965.

663. Wagener, H. P.: Arterioles of retina in toxemia of pregnancy. J.A.M.A. *101*:1380, 1933.

664. Wagener, H. P., and Hollenhorst, R. W.: The ocular lesions of temporal arteritis. Am. J. Ophthalmol. *45*:617, 1958.

665. Walsh, F. B.: Ocular importance of sarcoid; its relation to uveoparotid fever. Arch. Ophthalmol. *21*:421, 1939.

666. Walsh, F. B.: *Clinical Neuro-ophthalmology.* 2nd ed. Baltimore, Williams & Wilkins, 1957, p. 897.

667. Walsh, F. B., and Howard, J. E.: Conjunctival and corneal lesions in hypercalcemia. J. Clin. Endocrinol. *7*:644, 1947.

668. Walsh, F. B., Clark, D. B., Thompson, R. S., and Nicholsan, D. H.: Oral contraceptives and neuro-ophthalmologic interest. Arch. Ophthalmol. 74:628, 1965.
669. Walsh, F. G., and Hoyt, W. F.: Clinical Neuro-ophthalmology. 3rd ed. Baltimore, Williams & Wilkins, 1969, p. 72.
670. Walsh, T. J., Garden, J. W., and Gallagher, B.: Obliteration of retinal venous pulsations. Am. J. Ophthalmol. 67:954, 1969.
671. Weber, R. B., Daroff, R. B., and Mackey, E. A.: Pathology of oculomotor nerve palsy in diabetes. Neurology 20:835, 1970.
672. Webster, J. E., and Gurdjian, E. S.: Carotid artery compression as employed both in the past and in the present. J. Neurosurg. 14:372, 1958.
673. Webster, J. E., Gurdjian, E. S., and Martin, F. A.: Carotid artery occlusion. Neurology 6:491, 1956.
674. Weicksel, J.: Angiomatosis beziehungsweise Angiokeratosis universalis (eine sehr seltene Haut-Gefässerkrankung). Dtsch. Med. Wochenschr. 51:898, 1925.
675. Weigelin, E., and Lobstein, A.: Ophthalmodynamometrie. Basel, S. Karger, 1962.
676. Weigelin, E., and Putz, H.: Anticoagulantienbehandlung bei Venenthrombose der Netzhaut. Ber. Dtsch. Ophthalmol. Ges. 70:438, 1970.
677. Welch, R. B., and Goldberg, M. F.: Sickle-cell hemoglobin and its relation to fundus abnormality. Arch. Ophthalmol. 75:353, 1966.
678. Wells, R.: Microcirculation. In Conn, H. L., Jr., and Horwitz, O. (eds.): Cardiac and Vascular Diseases. Philadelphia, Lea & Febiger, 1971.
679. Wells, R. E., Schildkraut, E. R., and Edgerton, H. E.: Blood flow in the microvasculature of the conjunctiva of man. Science 151:995, 1966.
680. Wessing, A.: Fluoreszenzangiographie der retina. Stuttgart, Georg Thieme, 1968.
681. Wessing, A., and Meyer-Schwickerath, G.: Die Behandlung der Retinopathia diabetica mit Lichtkoagulation. Diabetologia 5:312, 1969.
682. Westby, R. K., and Dietrichson, P.: Insufficiency of the vertebral-basilar arterial system. With special reference to ocular symptoms and signs. Acta Ophthalmol. (Kbh.) 41:416, 1963.
683. White, P.: Childhood diabetes. Its course, and influence on the second and third generations. Diabetes 9:345, 1960.
684. Williams, I. M.: Intravascular changes in the retina during open-heart surgery. Lancet 2:688, 1971.
685. Wilson, R. S., and Ruiz, R. S.: Bilateral central retinal artery occlusion in homocystinuria. Arch. Ophthalmol. 82:267, 1969.
686. Wintrobe, M. M., and Buell, M. V.: Hyperproteinemia associated with multiple myeloma, with report of case in which extraordinary hyperproteinemia was associated with thrombosis of retinal veins and symptoms suggesting Raynaud's disease. Bull. Johns Hopkins Hosp. 52:156, 1933.
687. Wise, G. N.: Retinal microaneurysms. Arch. Ophthalmol. 57:151, 1957.
688. Wise, G. N.: The retinal venous obstructive syndrome. Eye Digest 2:4, 1958.
689. Wise, G. N., Dollery, C. T., and Henkind, P.: The Retinal Circulation. New York, Harper & Row, 1971.
690. Wolper, J., and Laibson, P. R.: Hereditary hemorrhagic telangiectasis (Rendu-Osler-Weber disease) with filamentary keratitis. Arch. Ophthalmol. 81:272, 1969.
691. Wolter, J. R.: Pathology of a cotton-wool spot. Am. J. Ophthalmol. 48:473, 1959.
692. Wolter, J. R.: Diabetic capillary microaneurysms of the retina. Arch. Ophthalmol. 65:847, 1961.
693. Wolter, J. R.: The nature of capillary microaneurysms in diabetic retinopathy. Diabetes 11:126, 1962.
694. Wolter, J. R.: The cytoid body reaction of the human retina. Trans. Am. Ophthalmol. Soc. 65:106, 1967.
695. Wolter, J. R.: Axonal enlargements in the nerve-fiber layer of the human retina. Am. J. Ophthalmol. 65:1, 1968.
696. Wolter, J. R., and Phillips, R. L.: Secondary glaucoma in cranial arteritis. Am. J. Ophthalmol. 59:625, 1965.
697. Wong, V. G., Schulman, J. D., and Seegmiller, J. E.: Conjunctival biopsy for the biochemical diagnosis of cystinosis. Am. J. Ophthalmol. 70:278, 1970.
698. Wood, F. A., and Toole, J. F.: Carotid artery occlusion and its diagnosis by ophthalmodynamometry. J.A.M.A. 165:1264, 1957.

699. Wray, S. H., and Cogan, D. G.: Unpublished.
700. Wright, J. C.: Angioid streaks in pituitary tumour. Br. J. Ophthalmol. 48:402, 1964.
701. Wybar, K. C.: Study of choroidal circulation of eye in man. J. Anat. 88:94, 1954.
702. Wybar, K. C.: Vascular anatomy of the choroid in relation to selective localization of ocular disease. Br. J. Ophthalmol. 38:513, 1954.
703. Yanoff, M.: Diabetic retinopathy. N. Engl. J. Med. 274:1344, 1966.
704. Yonechi, K., Yamada, N., Sato, N., and Chiba, M.: Fluorescence fundus angiography in sarcoidosis with special reference to perivasculitis. Excerp. Med. Ophthalmol. 25:6, 1971.
705. Zacharias, L.: Retrolental fibroplasia. (Letter). Am. J. Ophthalmol. 49:382, 1960.
706. Zimmerman, L. E.: Embolism of central retinal artery; secondary to myocardial infarction with mural thrombosis. Arch. Ophthalmol. 73:822, 1965.
707. Zimmerman, L. E., de Venecia, G., and Hamasaki, D. I.: Pathology of the optic nerve in experimental acute glaucoma. Invest. Ophthalmol. 6:109, 1967.
708. Zuidema, G. D., Burke, J. F., Villegas, A. H., and Scannell, J. G.: Surgery of atrial myxoma. N. Engl. J. Med. 264:1016, 1961.
709. Zweifach, P. H.: Moving retinal and choroidal emboli. Arch. Ophthalmol. 78:705, 1967.

INDEX

Note: Page numbers in *italic* indicate illustrations.

184 INDEX

Fundus sign(s) (*Continued*)
  significance of, cotton-wool spots, 44
    detachment of retina, 65
    diffuse opacity, 60
    exudates, 47
    hemorrhages, 50
    narrowing of arteries, 41
    optic atrophy, 62
    papilledema, 57
    vascular proliferative retinopathy,
     55

Gaucher's disease, diffuse retinal opacification in, 61
Glaucoma, and retinal vein occlusion, 130
  arterial pulsation in, 28
  congestion of retinal veins in, 42
  in sickle cell disease, 115
  100 day, of Coats, 128, 129
Grönblad-Strandberg syndrome, angioid streaks in, 97
Gunn's sign, 79

"Halo ensheathing," 43
Headache(s), cluster, 72
Heart disease, congenital, congestion of
    retinal veins in, 42
    tortuosity of retinal arteries in, 42
  rheumatic, emboli in, 120
    intracranial vascular accident in, 152
Hemangiomatosis, trigeminal, dilatation of conjunctival vessels in, 5
Hemianopia, 70, 70–72, 73
  bitemporal, causes of, 147
  differential diagnosis of, 151
  lesions of parietotemporal lobe and, 151, 154
  occipital lesions and, 150, 150, 154
Hemophilia, retinopathy with, 99
Hemorrhage(s), 50, 66
  angioid streaks and, 96
  flame-shaped, 50
  focally massive, 51, 51
  in fundus, 50
  in retinal vein occlusion, 127
  in sickle cell disease, 114
  involving conjunctiva, 9–12, 11, 12
  pre-retinal, 53, 53
  retinal, in diabetes, 90
  subarachnoid, 53, 54
  subhyaloid, 51
  subretinal, 53, 55
  vitreous, causes of, 53
    in diabetic retinopathy, 85, 85
  with tributary arterial occlusion, 52
Henle's fiber layer, 32
Herpes simplex, and primary vasculitis, 137

Homocystinuria, and occlusion of retinal vessels, 118
Horner's syndrome, with cluster headaches, 72
Hyperbetalipoproteinemia, arcus juvenilis in, 16
Hypercalcemia, band keratopathy with, 2, 2
Hypercholesteremia, arcus juvenilis in, 14, 15
  beading of retinal artery in, 95, 96
  signs of, in fundus, 93–95
Hyperglobulinemia, and retinal vein occlusion, 130
Hyperlipemia, lactescence of retinal vessels in, 93, 95
  signs of, in fundus, 93–95
Hypertension, cotton-wool spots in, 44, 45, 46, 75
  eclamptic, 76
  exudates in, 47
  flame-shaped hemorrhage in, 51
  narrowing of retinal arteries in, 41, 74, 75
  papilledema with, 58
  retinal vessels in, 76
  signs of, in fundus, 74–78, 100
  stages of, Keith-Wagener classification of, 77
  with carotid stenosis, 75
Hypotension, signs of, in fundus, 78, 101
Hypoxia, and blackouts, 68

Indocyanine, in fluoroangiography, 26
Inflammation, of eye, 3
Innominate steal syndrome, 114, 152
Iridocyclitis, inflammation in, 3
Irvine-Gass syndrome, 119

Jaundice, and yellow sclera, 1

Keith-Wagener classification, of hypertension, 77
Keratitis, inflammation in, 3
Keratopathy, band, with hypercalcemia, 2, 2

Lamina cribrosa, function of, 37
  in occlusion of retinal artery, 103
  in retinal vein obstruction, 52
Lead poisoning, angioid streaks in, 98
Leber's telangiectasis, exudates in, 47
Lesion(s), chorioretinal, 63, 67
Leukemia, congestion of retinal veins in, 4, 42
  retinopathy with, 99, 99
  Roth spots in, 52